FINDING MEANING *with* CHARLES

Gloria
My best to you & your future
life changes —

Brad C

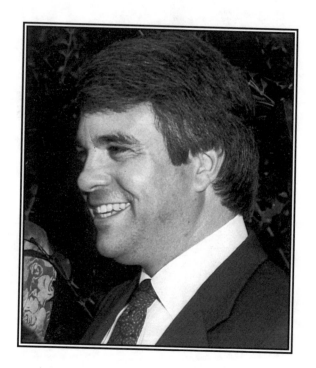

CHARLES EDMUNSON

FINDING MEANING
with CHARLES

*Caregiving with Love
Through a
Degenerative Disease*

Janet Edmunson

JME Insights
Danvers, Massachusetts
2006

"Five O'Clock World." Words and Music by Allen Reynolds © 1965 (Renewed 1993) SCREEN GEMS-EMI MUSIC INC. All rights reserved. International Copyright Secured. Used by Permission.

"Foolish Games." Word and music by Jewel Kilcher. © 1995 Wiggly Tooth Music. All rights controlled and administered by EMI April Music Inc. All Rights Reserved. International Copyright Secured. Used by Permission.

"My Heart Will Go On (Love Theme from 'Titanic')," from Paramount and Twentieth Century Fox Motion Picture TITANIC. Music by James Horner. Lyric by Will Jennings. Copyright © 1997 by Famous Music Corporation, Ensign Music Corporation, T.C.P. Music Publishing, Inc., Fox Film Music Corporatioin and Blue Sky Rider Songs. All Rights for Blue Sky Rider Songs Administered by Irving Music, Inc. International Copyright Secured. All Rights Reserved.

Letting Go: Morrie's Reflections on Living While Dying, Morrie Schwartz. New York: Walker & Company, 1996, p. 125.

Phenomenon, Gerald Di Pego. Touchstone Pictures, 1996.

JME Insights
Danvers, Massachusetts 01923
www.findingmeaningwithcharles.com

LCN: 2006903401
ISBN: 978-0-9778133-0-8

Cover design, book design and composition by The Quick Brown Fox
Edited by Katharine O'Moore-Klopf of KOK Edit (http://www.kokedit.com)
Copyedited by Melissa J. Hayes
Production Management by Jeremy Townsend, PublishingWorks Inc.
Printed in Canada

Caregiving is not a solo endeavor.

I dedicate this book to
all those who helped me
care for Charles—our families,
the nurses and doctors, friends,
and work colleagues.

None of us is as strong as all of us.

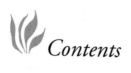 *Contents*

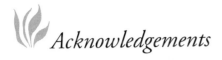 *Acknowledgements*

As Charles would always say, "The essence of life is relationships." My sincerest thanks to all who supported Charles and me during his illness, and for supporting me in writing this book.

Thanks for Your Graciousness:

✦ *Family*—for going above and beyond to help me and Charles in more ways than I can acknowledge here. Thank you Mom, Lois, Curt, Doug, Nancy, Barb, Jack, Sue, Fred, Carolyn, Tony, Ken, Shari, David, and Jayne.

✦ *Colleagues at Blue Cross Blue Shield of Massachusetts*—to my staff, whom I cannot thank enough for their support; to my leaders, who allowed my flexible working arrangements to give me time to write; and to my many friends who encouraged me.

✦ *Stacey and Joe Scala*—for providing the Big Yellow House on Prince Edward Island where I spent a week organizing my thoughts for the book, and for Stacey's regular back massages that released my pent-up tension.

✦ *June Sekera*—for providing direction for the book and also for allowing me to spend a week writing at her home overlooking the Cascade Mountains near Olympia and the Puget Sound.

✦ *Brenda Loube*—for allowing me to use her vacation home in St. Petersburg, Florida, to write for a week.

Thanks for Your Inspiration:

✦ *Beacon Roundtable Writing Group*—for the concrete suggestions you gave me. Thanks especially to Wendy Dodek, Suzanne Hanser, Steve Gordon, Susan Meyers, and Rosemary Walker.

✦ *Ken Edmunson*—for checking in on me regularly to make sure I was making progress.

✦ *Gibby Kinsey*—who while suffering with her own health issues, called Charles every week throughout his illness and supported me in my writing.

✦ *Kathy Edwards Elsaesser*—I fondly remember you drawing and me writing while sitting in front of beautiful sites on our trip to Budapest, Vienna, and Prague.

- *Corey Rosen*—who read an early draft and encouraged me to include more about Charles and me in the book.
- *Friends and Colleagues*—including Calvin Arey, Jean and Frank Boccelli, Michael Brower, Sharlet Cover, Charlie Derber, Arlene DiSalvo, Dick and Carol Duffy, Denise Jolicoeur, Debbie Jordan, Chris Moranetz, Melanie Nichol, Loren Rodgers, Julie Ross, Steve and Katie Sheppard, Bill Torbet, and Barbi White, who encouraged me when they read parts of the manuscript.
- *Maria Paige*—for reading an early draft of the manuscript and calling to tell me how compelling it was.

Thanks for Your Care:

- *Dr. Paula Ravin*—for working hard to help Charles with symptoms and an understanding of his disease.
- *Wayside Hospice, a program of Parmenter VNA & Community Care*— for Dianne Oelberger, our nurse, whose care and expertise got us through; for Judy Smith and Sue Anderson, who coordinated the volunteers; for Kathleen Heffernan, the social worker who helped me believe that I could make it; and to all of the volunteers—Lil Kelly, Bob Johnson, Maggie Taylor, Mike Toomey—and other staff members who became invaluable to Charles and me.
- *Dr. Michael Gamache, neuropsychologist*—who helped me understand the autopsy report, which released me from some overpowering concerns about Charles's behaviors.
- *All of Charles's aides.*

Thanks for Your Assistance:

- *Katharine O'Moore-Klopf, my editor*—who brought tremendous expertise to the writing process.
- *Jeremy Townsend, my publisher*—who made the book a reality.
- *Deidre Randall, my publicist*—who is working hard to tell others about this work.
- *Patty Marcille*—for editing early versions of the manuscript.

Thanks for Your Love:

- *Jim Landau*—for buoying me up when I doubted my writing ability. The e-mail you sent made me sob, but also gave me renewed strength to tackle writing with a fresh new enthusiasm. I love you, my husband and partner. I am so glad that the universe was gracious enough to bring me love twice in life.

At some time, everyone loses a loved one. Coldly, there is a time for everyone to go. Clearly, that was not the case for Charles. Thankfully, few people go through what you went through. Thankfully, you are caring enough to care about those people that will.

Look at all of the people that need your story. They need to know what it was like. What are you proud of? What would you have done differently? They want and deserve your story.

Would you not want everyone to know about how you came through with some strength? Is there a weakness of yours that you can share so others may know to watch for it? They want and deserve your story.

It must have been hard on your mother. This will be a hard, unwanted ordeal for every caring mother-in-law. What did she learn from Charles? What do you wish she had learned from Charles? They want and deserve your story.

How could your brother and sisters have continued to have joy in their lives when yours was turning so cold? What do you want them to learn from Charles? They want and deserve your story.

Any one that loses a loved one may find a new loved one. What do you want the new one to know about the past one? What do you want others to know about how to prepare for a new situation? They want and deserve your story.

You go, girl!

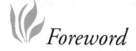

Foreword

I am honored to write about my experience of working with Charles and Janet Edmunson, but saddened by the realization that, years later, we have made little progress in diagnosing and treating most of the Parkinson's Plus syndromes. The publicity surrounding prominent public figures with Parkinson's disease has led to increased awareness of the personal toll of these disorders, and generated more dedicated research funds over the short term. Yet, many families still struggle with access to subspecialty care in neurology, and many say they need more time for effective communication with their doctors and other caregivers. There are only twenty fellowship programs in the entire USA dedicated to movement disorders (primarily Parkinsonian syndromes), and no certification or fiscal incentive to focus on clinical management of these diseases. The result is that few families can find the answers they need through the medical professionals they encounter.

There is a move in the international Movement Disorder Society and the American Academy of Neurology to advance the standards of care for patients with Parkinsonism through a formalized fellowship process, which would generate Medicare funds to support the programs. The process is tedious and requires encouragement by families of patients with Parkinsonian disorders, to let their physicians know that they need specialized care. This is not an affront to their local neurologists' knowledge or empathy, but rather an acknowledgment of the complexity of these diseases and the need for more integrated services.

Janet and Charles were able to maintain a quality of life at home right up to his peaceful passing. With many medical support services and community and church outreach, they had time to accept and adjust to Charles's disease even without a firm diagnosis. They sought a more definitive answer by donating Charles's brain to the Brain Tissue Resource Center, and planned for the process in advance. Finally, Janet has brought this book to fruition as a tribute to Charles and his determination to keep communicating with those around him. She loved him, cared for him, and honors him with her efforts to reach out to other families stricken with Parkinson's Plus syndromes.

I learned from Janet and Charles that we, as physicians, need to be humble when confronting indeterminate diagnoses and long disease processes that can follow an unpredictable course. "I don't know" is an important phrase to use while sharing in the patients' care with families. We can still be supportive and instrumental in coordinating services while questioning our own diagnoses, and awaiting the answers we may never find. I am always grateful when I receive notes from family members after they no longer come to my office, letting me know what happened to their loved ones, and how I helped them. I will continue to be optimistic about the clinical management of Parkinson's Plus patients because of this feedback, which reaffirms that the effort was worthwhile. Now, we must provide that same feedback to caregivers just beginning to learn about Parkinson's Plus syndromes—and Janet's book will help do just that.

—Paula D. Ravin, MD
Board Certified by the American Board of Psychiatry and Neurology
Associate Professor of UMass Medical School
Fellowship—National Institutes of Health

INTRODUCTION

It wasn't until about the third year of Charles's disease that the Serenity Prayer had its greatest impact on me. But I have always loved it, and it means the most to me when I am going through tough times: " . . . grant me the *serenity to accept* the things I cannot change, courage to change the things I can, and wisdom to know the difference."

I have really latched onto the concept of "accepting the things I cannot change." Though we tried to fight it, Charles's disease was going to take away his abilities, and eventually, his life. Our choice was to accept that or deny it.

I don't know for sure what Charles's choice was. He was determined not to let the disease change his life and goals. He tried hard to keep contributing as best he could. That was how Charles tackled everything in life. He denied the obstacle and set out to conquer it. He wouldn't succumb. He fought all the way to the end. Is that acceptance or denial?

I, however, consciously chose to accept it and make the most of it.

My greatest learning through this experience came when Charles and I attended the Mind/Body Medical Institute program which at the time was held at Beth Israel Deaconess Hospital in Boston. The instructor, Peg, talked about acceptance, explaining that the way to accept the things that we have no control over, such as an illness, is to make meaning out of it. Wow! Make meaning out of it! Her explanation suddenly allowed me to consciously look at what Charles and I were going through and identify where it helped us grow and where it allowed us to have an impact on others that we wouldn't have had without the adversity of his disease.

Taking a proactive approach to making meaning out of our situation helped me to positively focus on the opportunities and not plunge into depression. I was determined to help Charles reach whatever potential his life could give. And I was amazed to see how Charles became even more influential—even after he could no longer talk. As a caregiver, I found it important to focus on this greater purpose. My goal for caregiving went beyond making sure Charles was safe and physically cared for. I wanted to ensure that he still lived life to the fullest—to whatever degree the disease would allow.

Accepting Charles's disease and making meaning out of it didn't mean that we didn't feel pain. Coping with this type of degeneration was difficult physically and emotionally for Charles, the person with the disease, as well as for me, the caregiver. We faced many trials—some successfully, others not. But we both became better people through experiencing his disease.

M. Scott Peck starts his book *The Road Less Traveled* with the sentence "Life is difficult." He goes on to explain that once we accept this, we can begin to make the most of life. Charles and I had discussed this concept a number of times when we faced problems at work or with other people. The misfortune of his disease forced us to face our greatest life difficulty, truly testing our ability to accept adversity and then move on.

I don't know of anyone who expressed this thought better than Viktor Frankl in his book *Man's Search for Meaning*. Frankl survived the atrocities and indignities of a concentration camp in World War II. He realized there that to renew our inner strength, we need to have a future goal. He quoted Nietzsche's words, "He who has a why to live for can bear with almost any how." I found that "finding meaning" is a way to define the why. The act of looking for and finding meaning in Charles's disease focused and empowered me.

I hope that this book will encourage you to find and make meaning out of your life's tragedies. I've included Caregiving Affirmations in each chapter. You may find some of these to be especially inspiring to you. Hang on to them, repeat them, and let them focus you on building the strength you need.

1

❧

1995: As if Life Were Still Normal

Helping Charles Face His Symptoms

"I seem to have problems when I go down stairs. And I struggle to make my hand meet a cashier's when getting change," Charles reluctantly admitted. But he didn't volunteer this information until I brought up the topic of his disturbing symptoms.

I had begun to notice some startling physical changes in him. For example, he seemed uptight when driving—sitting forward, clutching the steering wheel tightly, looking not at all confident.

In the summer of 1995, happily married and enjoying our fast-paced lifestyle of hard work and lots of travel, we visited my parents in Florida especially to see my dad, who had cancer of the larynx. After two operations and chemotherapy, it had spread to his lungs in the late stage.

The first night of our visit, Charles wobbled unsteadily while getting down onto the mattress we had placed on the floor from the pullout bed. After I'd observed his driving posture, this unsteadiness made me feel sure something was wrong. But I didn't know how to approach him. For some reason, I struggled with how to initiate this conversation. Finally I said, in as tender a voice as I could, "Charles, why are you so unsteady? Is something wrong?"

Reluctantly, he admitted, "I'm beginning to think so. I just kept hoping it would go away." Then he shared with me the difficulties he'd been experiencing recently.

I don't know how long Charles would have waited, if I hadn't asked, before confessing his problem. In some ways, he was a very private person. And I can't even imagine how it felt to be in his shoes, not having complete control of his body. But I think that finally admitting his difficulties brought him some comfort and relief.

Caregiving Affirmation:
Approach your loved one sympathetically.
A gentle approach can bring breakthrough communication.

Charles later told me that he first noticed a problem while attending the ESOP (Employee Stock Ownership Plan) Association conference earlier that year, in May. The association had been filming a video in Washington, D.C. "I kept stumbling going up and down the stairs of the Capitol building, and I wasn't able to keep up with the others," Charles explained.

Because Charles's dad, Ralph, had Parkinson's disease, I first jumped to the conclusion that Charles had the same condition. But their symptoms differed. Ralph's disease first affected his hands, making typing difficult. Then he began to shuffle when he walked. Though Charles and I both tried to hide it, fear crept over us as we imagined the worst possible scenario. He was only forty-five, and his first symptoms had appeared so much earlier than his dad's had. Would the disease progress more quickly and be more severe for Charles because of his younger age?

When I worked as the wellness manager for Georgia-Pacific Corporation a few years earlier, one of the lawyers, probably in his forties, had Parkinson's. Over a few short years, I watched it dramatically affect his gait and speech. The last I knew, he was on disability and getting experimental treatments.

I had no idea that what Charles had could actually be something even worse.

Needing an Active Role in Treatment

This wasn't Charles's first medical crisis.

Here again, he followed in his dad's footsteps.

His dad had had triple-bypass heart surgery at the age of sixty. When Charles was only forty-three, he agreed to have an angioplasty. Surgeons threaded a tiny tube from the right side of his groin all the way up to his heart. Once they found the blockage, they pumped air into a small balloon at the end of the tube to open up the heart's artery. Afterward, Charles grinned with glee, the before and after pictures of his arteries in hand. "I could watch the entire procedure on the monitors," he said. "I could see everything they did. But boy, did it hurt when they pumped the balloon. What a terrible squeezing pain! Thank goodness it didn't last long. That must be what a heart attack feels like."

The angioplasty came after about ten years of off-and-on chest pain while Charles jogged. During that time, mostly when we lived in Atlanta, Charles had had exercise stress tests, echocardiograms, and numerous visits to cardiologists. None of the test results were conclusive; most were normal. Only the echocardiogram turned out a little iffy, not serious enough to warrant an official diagnosis of heart disease.

It wasn't until we had moved back to the Boston area in the early 1990s that Charles started having chest pain even when just walking. His new primary care doctor took a proactive approach, giving him some cholesterol and heart function medications. If these didn't work, we would then consider arteriography to determine whether any of Charles's arteries needed another procedure to unclog them. In an arteriogram, a doctor looks at the heart's arteries through a probe also threaded from the groin.

When the medications didn't relieve the pain, we decided that Charles should undergo arteriography. It showed a blockage of more than 90 percent in the circumflex artery of his heart. This somewhat minor branch of the coronary artery feeds a less critical part of the heart. Thankfully, the doctors discovered only minimal blockage in the "widowmaker" artery—the main artery that feeds the left ventricle, the powerful part of the heart that pumps blood to the entire body.

After receiving these results, we decided to just continue the medication therapy. A fully blocked circumflex artery probably wouldn't kill him, so it seemed worth the risk.

Unfortunately, the medications still didn't remove the pain.

"I'm having chest pains," Charles confessed one evening, just before bed. "And they're getting more severe." We gave him the recommended three spaced-out doses of nitroglycerine under his tongue, but that didn't help, so we went to Boston to Brigham and Women's Hospital. He was immediately admitted, and then before we knew it, the angioplasty was complete.

All of this taught me that one of my roles was to urge Charles to get appropriate medical help. Charles was inclined to procrastinate and hope that things would improve on their own—but he didn't seem to mind my encouraging him to see a doctor or to go to the emergency room if something really seemed to be wrong.

It turned out that another of my roles during Charles's mystery condition was accompanying him to his doctor appointments. Because the chest pain represented a crisis, I accompanied Charles on most of the doctor visits. But once the crisis was over, Charles went to all the follow-up appointments alone.

By the time Charles's neurological symptoms appeared, he'd been quite healthy and free of heart disease symptoms. And because I didn't even imagine that these symptoms could spell such doom, I didn't go with him on the initial visits to his primary care doctor or to his first consult with the neurologist, Dr. Paula Ravin.

Because I hadn't participated in the early physician visits about this new problem, I understood the issues only through the filter of Charles's explanation. And justifiably, he never seemed to remember all of the details. It's hard for a patient to absorb a lot of new information well enough to be able to repeat it back to someone else. I learned quickly that I had to commit to attending every appointment with Charles so that he could get the best possible care.

Caregiving Affirmation:
Engage actively with doctors to enhance your loved one's care.

A SPECIAL CONNECTION

I wanted Charles to have top-notch care because he had been so special to me for such a long time, since we were both in our late twenties.

I first saw him—before I actually met him—in the late 1970s at the nondenominational Christian church I attended in Wakefield, Massachusetts. The small congregation of fewer than a hundred people met on the second floor of a local municipal building. Sitting on a metal folding chair, I noticed a visitor walk in a bit late and take a seat on the other side of the cramped hall. He wore a camel-colored corduroy suit jacket with suede patches at the elbows. He looked to be about my age. I wondered if this cute, brown-haired man with sparkling brown eyes could be single. I didn't get a chance to meet him—or maybe it was just that I was too shy to take the chance to introduce myself. But later I asked some friends at the church if they remembered the visitor and knew who he was.

"That was Charles Edmunson," Randall replied. "I went to college with him in Florida. He's in graduate school here at Boston University, and he's separated from his wife."

Oh well, I thought, and gave up on the passing fantasy of a potential boyfriend. I figured that if he was only separated, he wasn't ready yet for a new relationship. And it went against my beliefs to date someone still involved in a marriage.

A year or two later, Charles showed up at church again. He was shorter than I remembered but still just as cute, though now sporting a full beard and mustache. At around five foot four, I was nearly his height; he stood at five foot six. Fitting in with the fashions of the time, I had long blonde hair—soon to be permed and cut to have bangs—that framed my oval face and teal-blue eyes. I wore a pair of light-blue corduroy jeans and a sweater, my typical casual wear at that age.

After the service, he attended the singles get-together at my friend Jean's apartment. We happened to drift together, and soon started a deep philosophical and spiritual discussion, the first of many we would share over time.

"Why do you believe as strongly as you do in God?" Charles asked. I passionately explained all the reasons I felt that I had seen God working in my life.

During our conversation, I learned that he was teaching philosophy part-time at the University of Massachusetts Boston and Bridgewater State College, as well as at Bridgewater State Prison. And he worked part-time at a manufacturing company called Web Converting, whose founder was a strong Christian. He told me that he visited the church I attended for socializing, not necessarily because he was searching spiritually.

Over the next few months, I'd see Charles occasionally at church services. And often when the church had a special event, Charles would attend. Each time, we'd end up together, continuing our deep and intense conversation about faith and philosophy. Over time, I learned that Charles had studied to be a minister at Florida College, the extremely fundamentalist Church of Christ school in Tampa. That was where he had also met a couple of the people who now attended the Wakefield church with me.

While he was still in high school, Charles traveled great distances to preach at small, rural churches in Arkansas that couldn't afford a full-time minister. He found tremendous fulfillment at that early age in using his gift for speaking and his passionate religious beliefs.

At Florida College, Charles married one of his classmates. They soon moved to Jackson, Mississippi, where he had been offered a preaching job, and he began taking graduate classes in philosophy. Just a year later, Charles and his wife moved back to Tampa, where he continued his philosophy studies at the University of South Florida to earn the first of two master's degrees. It was at that point, Charles said, that he lost his faith.

"What do you mean, you lost your faith?" I asked.

"I became an agnostic," Charles replied. "The only thing I know is that I can't know if there is a God." Circumstances at the churches he attended, along with his philosophy studies, led him to that point, which he said devastated his relationship with his wife and derailed his lifelong dream of becoming a minister. "How could I keep preaching if I no longer believed?" he asked.

At that time, my faith was my life. I clearly fit the definition of a born-again Christian. I didn't just go to church; I asked God every day to help me do His will. I saw my life as living evangelism—helping others experience the love of God—so part of my attraction to Charles came from my desire to help him find God again.

But part of it was also his strong personal magnetism. At a good-bye party for the minister of the Wakefield church, Charles and I had another engaging conversation. Within a week, I got my first phone call from him. He asked me to dinner. Naively thinking that we could keep our relationship at the level of friendship alone, I accepted. Despite my attraction to him, I was truly enjoying our friendship and wanted to keep it just the way it was.

We continued to get together quite regularly, always discussing faith and life. In one of our early conversations, Charles asked, "If God is God, why would He make it so hard for us to believe and know His reality? Why does God hide Himself? Janet, I think that if God called me into judgment, I would claim that *He* was unfair."

"Although I have had doubts, and still do," I responded, "I have known God in my inner heart. But only to the extent that He at times has revealed Himself to me—only in my asking and seeking, not in my doing anything."

Early in our relationship, Charles jotted down his gnawing thoughts, which I later found in a folder:

I am to the point where I want to believe. And sometimes I feel that I will believe; my defenses are down; my heart is bare. But I am aware of so many questions: Will God give me no peace about them? Must each one be a needle in my flesh? Sometimes it fits. Maybe even I am beginning to know. Lord, give me courage.

Every week I seem to cross the universe. From unbelief, out-right skepticism, to bewilderment, back to incredulity, slipping toward hope, dreaming of certainty. How vast is the territory within!

Our stimulating and thoughtful conversations captivated both of us, further deepening our friendship.

Then one night, he unexpectedly kissed me. Startled, I froze, then said, "Good night," and quickly raced up the stairs into the apartment that I shared with two other roommates. Charles would later say that I reacted like a scared rabbit—and I guess I did. Intellectually, I saw him as a friend, but emotionally, I was falling in love with him.

We began to explore our relationship romantically while still continuing our spiritual and philosophical discussions. The notes in his folder confirmed that he was falling for me:

Janet—

Activities and companionship—

Hungry to get to know you; time spent passively watching a movie is wasted. I scarcely know what I'm eating when I'm with you.

On the other hand, I'm surprised that we never run out of things to say to each other. Most of the time I feel empty and shallow—as if my soul could be plumbed by an insightful being within a few minutes.

But we are doing more than communicating information. I've noticed that by the end of our evenings together, what we are saying does not seem to matter. We are touching, emotionally, even spiritually. We are communicating affection, compassion, and reaching for intimacy. Such communication transcends ideas.

When I want too much for you to like me, I am not myself. And you can't know me. That *is the curse of romance.*

I finally became convinced that Charles was right for me when he had us define our values. I had always expected to marry a Christian believer, so I wouldn't succumb and allow our relationship to grow until I was sure that he was right for me despite his lapsed faith. "Write a list of all the things you value," he instructed me. He wrote his own list—and then we matched them together. Almost all of the values, such as helping others, and even the pursuit of a better understanding of faith, appeared on both lists. I was convinced that we had key core values in common.

We were married in September 1980 at a quaint historic building in Lynnfield, Massachusetts, about a year and a half after our first date.

Caregiving Affirmation:
Reflect on your special relationship for inspiration
when life gets overwhelming.

SEARCHING FOR A DIAGNOSIS

"Well, what did she say?" I asked Charles as soon as he was back home from his first visit with the neurologist.

"It could be Parkinson's, but she doesn't think so. She had some other suggestions that didn't sound much better. She suspects it is a movement disorder like Parkinson's." That was about all that Charles could remember of what Dr. Ravin had said.

Then he plopped his briefcase onto the kitchen counter and pulled out a wad of papers. "She gave me this video and brochure on Parkinson's disease." Then he showed me articles on multiple system atrophy (MSA), a condition about which Dr. Ravin had personally conducted research, and a newsletter on progressive supranuclear palsy (PSP) from the Society for PSP (http://www.psp.org). "She gave me these two pills, too. They apparently are superantioxidants that are supposed to slow down the progression of my symptoms," he said.

Charles seemed annoyed that the doctor couldn't pin down this disease more fully. "She doesn't know exactly what it is," he said, totally frustrated. And even with my health background, I was hearing the names of these rare diseases for the first time. I felt lost, not knowing what to do next, or how to comfort him in this new journey full of unknowns. All we could do was hug each other and cry.

In a follow-up visit with Dr. Ravin, we learned that another potential explanation for Charles's symptoms could be a disease in this same family of movement disorders, called cortical basal ganglionic degeneration (CBGD). MSA, PSP, and CBGD fall into the Parkinson family of disorders that neurologists called Parkinson-plus. I had heard about Parkinson's before, but not all of these others. Could there really be so many different movement disorders? Their names alone sounded awful and complicated. What could they be? What would they mean for Charles? He needed to know.

Dr. Ravin was sure, after that first examination, that Charles had a developing neurological condition. The tough job was for her to determine which class of disease he had, so that she could find appropriate treatments. Until she could make an exact diagnosis, all the medicines she prescribed would be merely educated guesses. If they worked, great; if not, she would try another. Neurological diseases produce odd symptoms. The difficulty in narrowing the diagnosis was that symptoms of neurological diseases unfold over time, and the same symptoms can appear in a number of them. It might be years, if at all, before enough symptoms emerged to clearly point to a true diagnosis.

It was the not knowing that slowly started to consume Charles. "I need to know so that I can feel sure I'm doing all I can to beat this disease," he said. We decided that if the doctors couldn't tell him, we would do our own research.

Totally frazzled at my new job, I felt overwhelmed thinking of the time needed to conduct this research, as well as keep up with doctor visits. How could I squeeze in a half day here and there to go with Charles to the doctor? I worked in Boston, but Charles's doctors were in Worcester, about forty-five minutes away. Every visit seemed to take at least two hours, not including the long time spent in the waiting room. And how could I find time to look for more specialists and prepare for future unknown demands of caregiving?

I felt overwhelmed thinking of the level of effort portrayed by family members in the movie *Lorenzo's Oil,* reading volumes of journal articles and books to try to discover solutions for their loved one's unique disorder. I didn't think I could do that. Guilt crept in and began to haunt me. Charles struggled, too, with having time to cope with his nameless condition. It was hard for both of us to accept that there is never a good time to face the trauma of a major disease. But because we had to, Charles and I squeezed in time to do the homework that would help us begin to understand all the potential diagnoses.

Caregiving Affirmation:
If you have the time and energy to do even a little research,
you and your loved one may feel a welcome sense of control
over the chaos of disease.

TACKLING THE BOSTON PUBLIC LIBRARY

I hadn't been in the massive Boston Public Library since working on a high school term paper in the late 1960s. But now we needed the best library possible to educate ourselves on neurological diseases. We found the medical area deep in the bowels of the building.

Neurological textbooks provided the best summaries for us; but I soon found that even with my master's degree in health promotion, many of the neurological terms we came across were foreign to me—or I had forgotten them. I struggled to decipher the meanings of the terms for symptoms Charles might eventually have: *apraxia, dystonia, bradykinesia, dysphagia, bradyphrenia.* At least I understood *rigidity, apathy, tremor, dementia,* and *depression.* Some of the books gave hints as to what the difficult words meant, but for others I had to ask Dr. Ravin.

When it came to the causes for these Parkinson-plus diseases, though, all of the books were very clear: unknown! Of course, they discussed theories, and they outlined potential treatments—mostly medications that have been successful with Parkinson's. But for the rare diseases that Charles might have—PSP, MSA, and CBGD— these medications have been largely ineffective.

After making copies of some textbook chapters, we asked a librarian for help in conducting a search on MEDLINE (http://www.ncbi.nlm.nih.gov/entrez/query.fcgi), the U.S. National Library of Medicine's online database of millions of references to journal articles in the life sciences. Surprisingly, we found relatively few articles on these Parkinson-like diseases. And the ones we found were even more difficult to understand than the textbooks.

Our First Time Online
At that point, I had had minimal experience with the Internet, but friends and colleagues praised the vast information that was beginning to emerge there, so Charles and I went to my office one Saturday afternoon to give it a try. We found the Web sites for the Society for PSP and a British association dealing with PSP. We also found a few posts from people asking questions or giving answers.

Some of the most important information we discovered came from the Web site of the National Institutes of Health (NIH; http://www.nih.gov). The divisions of the National Institute of Neurological Disorders and Stroke (http://www.ninds.nih.gov) and the National Organization for Rare Disorders (http://www.rarediseases.org) were conducting research on these conditions, so we obtained the appropriate names, phone numbers, and addresses for follow-up.

Other Helpful Resources
The Society for PSP quickly became our most valuable resource. For a small membership fee, we joined immediately. We weren't certain that Charles had PSP, but the symptoms sounded very similar— problems with eye movements and body rigidity. We found the practical tips in the group's newsletter extremely helpful, and the research

summaries included studies for many of Charles's potential diagnoses, not just PSP. And the pamphlets helped us understand the common symptoms of many of these diseases. As the years went on, the newly organized society matured greatly and became a tremendous support for us.

A colleague told me about Planetree Health and Healing Library (www.myhealthandhealing.org), an organization in California connected with the Institute for Health & Healing and the California Pacific Medical Center that conducted in-depth MEDLINE searches for a fee. I ordered searches on PSP and CBGD. From the information we had found so far, Charles's symptoms seemed to fit most with these two diseases. Though most of the information in the articles sent by Planetree was incomprehensible to me, I did pick up some nuances that added to my overall understanding.

Our research had now begun in earnest. Would we learn anything that would be truly helpful to us as we continued on our journey?

AWFUL NEWS UNCOVERED

Charles had begun to struggle to get his eyes to follow a line of text, so I would read aloud to him the articles and chapters from textbooks we had photocopied. And because we led a full life, I would read these to him in the oddest places, such as sitting on a blanket at an outdoor Boston Pops concert, and when enjoying frozen yogurt at a local shop. As usual, we were making the most of our time by doing two things at once.

One of my clearest memories of that time is of the two of us sitting in the pink booth at our favorite frozen-yogurt parlor, devouring our daily frozen yogurt. Between bites of the scrumptious chocolate treat, I read to Charles the text we had copied from the neurology books at the Boston Public Library. The PSP information I read to him was depressing, but the CBGD details were even worse: The physical decline for those who have it progresses faster—and with more debilitating symptoms.

As I read, I came to a prediction of the life expectancy for those with CBGD: "The course is slowly progressive and ends fatally in five to ten years." Even though the shocking words shouted in my head, I kept reading without a pause, hoping nervously that Charles didn't catch them. He didn't wince or mention it, so I assumed that he didn't hear or understand. But the words unraveled me, and I never brought it up again.

I'm thankful that Charles seemed to predominantly hear the positive side of the literature. For instance, he was very comforted by a sentence from the PSP brochure that said that "although PSP gets progressively worse, no one dies from PSP itself." Later it said that "most PSP patients live well into their seventies and beyond." But that doesn't give a clear picture: Most people don't develop PSP until they are in their sixties. That would still leave a life expectancy as short as seven to ten years. But to Charles at age forty-five, living into his seventies sounded great! He hoped for that, just as I wished for as much time with him as possible.

Charles feared the cognitive symptoms most. He desperately didn't want to lose his intellect and mental capacity. Unfortunately, at least mild dementia occurs with most of the Parkinson-plus diseases. It begins earliest with CBGD, often starting with slowed mental responses—taking more time than usual to answer a question or synthesize information. And along with dementia, changes in personality sometimes appear, such as increased irritability and loss of interest in activities that once brought pleasure.

PSP and CBGD eventually affect the brain's control of eye movement. This leads to loss of balance while walking, and subsequently, falls. Stiff muscles, more common in CBGD, further impact the patient's ability to walk and move. Down the line, the patient has difficulty reading and driving a car.

Additionally, patients with CBGD find it hard to direct voluntary movements, affecting their ability to write, among other things. This might be why Charles struggled to make his hand meet those of cashiers when exchanging money. And CBGD can produce other odd symptoms, such as an arm drifting up into an unnatural position.

Later in the course of these diseases, speech and swallowing problems often occur as the part of the brain controlling them is affected. Speech can slow and then become slurred, until eventually, it is completely gone. Problems with swallowing can cause aspiration, which is when food and liquids slip into the lungs. Aspiration can lead to pneumonia, which often ultimately kills people with these diseases.

PSP was discovered only as recently as 1964. Add the rarity of all these diseases, and it's easy to see why they are often misdiagnosed as Parkinson's, or sometimes, Alzheimer's.

We found little good news in our research on PSP, CBGD, and MSA, and certainly no clarity yet on which disease Charles actually had. We were in shock that this was happening to him, and feared where it would lead. But we now started hoping that what he had was PSP, as it seemed the mildest of all of these disastrous options.

Caregiving Affirmation:
It's normal to feel shocked when you learn about the severity
of a neurodegenerative disease.

WHAT COULD HAVE CAUSED IT?

Whenever I talk to someone about Charles's disease, the question of what could have caused it almost always comes up. Charles and I were curious to know why his body was succumbing to this terrible deterioration. Maybe if we knew why, we could find something to slow it down or change its course. If we knew why, maybe it wouldn't seem so frightening. We had to look for a cause, even though it was unlikely that we could change the course of the disease.

Most of our doctors didn't even try to understand the causes. They focused on the diagnoses and treatments. And unfortunately, scientific researchers didn't have the answers—although theories abounded.

For Charles, the potential contributors seemed endless.

The most obvious was his family history of neurological disease. His father had Parkinson's, and his mother had Alzheimer's disease. These weren't what Charles had, but could he have inherited some sort of neurological weakness from his parents?

The neurologists always asked if Charles had had any significant chemical exposure in his life. He could think of a couple of potential culprits. When he was in college, he worked during one summer for plumbers. He remembered being sick from chemical fumes for a couple of days after spending time in a ditch, installing PVC pipe. Other summers, he worked for masons, but that seemed less of a potential offender, as fewer chemicals would have been used. In his work at Web Industries (formerly known as Web Converting) as an adult, he was exposed to the dust from various types of plastic, film, paper, and metal products. With a potential neurological weakness, could any of those materials have made him vulnerable?

Maybe his illness was caused by the heart disease he'd developed at an early age—perhaps it had weakened his neurological system? If not the heart disease itself, maybe it was the high doses of niacin that Charles took to raise his pitifully low levels of HDL (high-density lipoprotein, or "good") cholesterol. Niacin affects the central nervous system, so that seemed to be a plausible theory. Some research has shown that there is a higher incidence of dementia, decreased cognitive functioning, and emotional apathy among people who have undergone bypass surgery. Maybe Charles's angioplasty had triggered the neurological problems.

Being an "all or nothing" person, Charles had drastically changed his diet on learning about his blocked arteries when he underwent arteriography. He had already modified his diet to include the typical low-fat choices—more chicken instead of meat, and lower-fat snacks and treats—but now he was going to eat hardly any fat at all. He strictly adhered to a very low-fat diet, with chicken and four low-fat Healthy Choice sandwich cookies as his only sources of fat. Everything else he ate was nearly fat-free—items such as bagels, cereal, juice, fruit, vegetables, pasta, vegetarian chili, and frozen yogurt. Our brains need fat to help them function properly; could this extreme low-fat diet have had a deleterious effect on his brain?

As far as diet went, Charles also drank more than the average number of diet sodas each day. When I first met him, he was hooked on Mountain Dew, which has a high caffeine content. Then he switched to Coca-Cola. Once he started to try to lose weight, he switched to diet drinks, which contained NutraSweet. People at

Charles's office often commented to me that he would have a diet soda at his desk all day long. What impact, if any, could the NutraSweet have had on his neurological problems?

When I met Charles, he had never needed a dental filling. But he developed gum disease early on, at about the age of forty. It wasn't for lack of brushing his teeth. Every night, Charles scrubbed back and forth for at least ten minutes. But even though he spent lots of time brushing, he didn't brush in the proper way to remove the plaque. Recent scientific studies have shown an association between gum disease and heart disease. Could the bacteria growing so close to the brain have caused any of his problems?

Before his neurological symptoms started, ticks had bitten him a couple of times near his groin after he moved air conditioners from the dirt section of basement in our Victorian house into the bedroom windows. What role could the tick bites have played?

Prior to his disease, Charles traveled to a few foreign countries—China, Thailand, Hungary, and Japan. Could something he had eaten or breathed have had a bad effect on his brain? New research would later show that a plant in Guam might be causing a similar disease among the natives there.

A variety of sleep issues also raised my suspicions. I found it curious that Charles never remembered his dreams. On reflection, he had no recollection of any dreams—ever. Also, all throughout his thirties, when we slept together, Charles slept on his right side every night, never turning over to his left. Oddly, I remember discussing this with him at the time and warning that it might have an impact on his brain, although I doubted it really would. What a strange premonition of the brain disorder that would eventually affect him.

When Charles was quite heavy a few years before his neurological symptoms appeared, I believed he had sleep apnea. This is a serious condition in which a person stops breathing while sleeping and then suddenly gasps for air. I witnessed this night after night when he was overweight. His doctor at the time encouraged him to have a sleep test which he never took the time to get. And this condition was suspected during one of his hospitalizations later in his disease.

Recent research has linked this condition with heart disease and other problems. Though it went away when he lost weight, could it still have had a connection to his disease?

Once we moved back to Boston, when Charles worked at the Web Industries corporate headquarters, Charles used his car phone pretty extensively when traveling to and from work. Will we ever know whether cell phones and their precursors have a harmful effect on the brain?

Some of the research we read theorized that these types of diseases could be caused by a yet-to-be discovered virus. Reading that just prompted more questions. When could he have been exposed to the virus? How did the virus enter into his body? Why did the virus affect Charles and not me?

Exploring these theories together helped satisfy our need to understand all that we possibly could about this disease. No matter how much we speculated, though, we would never know the actual cause of his neurological disease. And with so many potential causes, it's no wonder science hasn't figured it out yet either.

Caregiving Affirmation:
Explore the causes of the condition together to gain understanding.

IMMERSED IN OUR PASSIONS AND CAREERS

Because we were both intense people, Charles and I worked with passion and commitment on the projects we believed in.

When Charles's neurological symptoms first started to appear in May, I had been at my new job at Blue Cross Blue Shield of Massachusetts only three months. I found meaning in my work as manager of the Prevention and Wellness Department. We encouraged Blue Cross members to get preventive screening tests, supported physicians in talking to their patients about prevention, and assisted companies in offering health promotion programs for their employees. And with a new and growing staff, I also took my job of employee development seriously. I wanted to mentor them both in their jobs and as people. I immersed myself in all the wonderful challenges my new job afforded. It took some time for me to hire enough people to share the increasing workload, so initially, much of the department's work fell to me. I worked seventy or more hours a week to just barely keep up. But that didn't matter; I loved it.

Charles was too busy changing the world, his workaholic style driving him into activities across the globe. As vice president for manufacturing for Web Industries' six plants across the United States, he spent hours each day taking care of his employees—calling them, visiting them, and mentoring them.

Beyond Web, he had become increasingly involved in the national ESOP Association, which promotes employee ownership of companies. He and his colleague Dick led the first-ever strategic planning process at the association, bringing the people-centered focus of employee ownership to the forefront, instead of just as it related to financial issues.

"Too many people are selling their lives for a paycheck," Charles would say. To him, employee ownership—in which the profits of a company go to its employees—created the structure that helped people find meaning in their jobs. Employee owners worked for themselves as well as for the company. The more efficient they were, the more the company would benefit and the more financial opportunity each employee would then have. Employee ownership synchronized perfectly with Charles's philosophy of the common good. Even as a young master's degree student in philosophy at Florida State University, he wrote his thesis on "ethical roots of Marxism."

Highly sought after as a speaker, Charles frequently traveled across the United States to speak to groups—and had just begun to travel abroad for international speaking engagements. He relished those opportunities to promote employee ownership and participatory management styles.

Life was moving along at a frenetic pace for both of us. But Charles had never done anything at a leisurely pace or in a half-hearted manner.

When Charles and I first met, he was working part time at Web Converting's manufacturing plant in Framingham, Massachusetts, the only location for the company at the time. This job helped support him while he worked on his doctoral degree in philosophy at Boston University. His job at Web was as a packer, putting the finished product into boxes for shipping. In time, he moved up to machine operator.

He was also teaching introductory philosophy courses at the University of Massachusetts Boston, at Bridgewater State College, and at Bridgewater State Prison. From the little bit he told me about these classes, I gather that he was a stimulating teacher, using creative techniques to get students to think for themselves.

But Charles became enamored of the people-centered philosophy of Web's founder. While we dated, he decided to build a career at Web instead of finishing his doctoral degree, not able to imagine himself teaching Philosophy 101 for many years to come. He wanted more options than the few he saw for philosophy graduates. Once he started full-time at Web, he quickly advanced to night shift supervisor, managing a team running the various machines.

Then shortly after we married, Web selected Charles to join the management team as sales manager, launching a new plant in Atlanta. With no formal business education or background, Charles used his instincts to help him progress. Initially, his dedication, loyalty, and intellect helped him succeed in sales. Soon Web promoted him to general manager.

As general manager, Charles refined his skills. He wanted his plant to be special. He showed tremendous care for his employees, listening to their needs, helping them with the dirty work on overtime shifts when the business was bustling, and being present for them when a crisis arose, such as staying with an employee in the emergency room when he was injured on the job. In many ways, Charles's job was his life. It gave him the opportunity to make a difference in people's lives and help them find meaning. He had developed a compassionate leadership style that made employees feel good about themselves and their contribution to their jobs.

"I frequently came away from spending time with Charles feeling more confident and excited about the future for both myself and the company," one of the sales managers told me. "By his actions, Charles reminded me that people always come first," said the management quality representative at one of Web's plants. An administrative assistant once said to Charles, "Your special gift to me has always been the way you see the person I want to be. Whenever you are near, I get a transfusion of confidence and self-esteem." And one of the machine operators said, "Charles gave me the initiative to do things I don't think were possible. Things that I thought were out of my grasp, he showed me were in my grasp."

And his approach worked. The Atlanta plant was quickly becoming the most profitable of the Web facilities.

Because he hadn't had formal education in business, though, Charles doubted his natural expertise. With the encouragement and support of the company, he joined the executive MBA program at Georgia State University. "After you have your degree," Bob Fulton, the company's founder and CEO, said, "I'd like to bring you back to Boston in a corporate capacity." So in September 1990, with his second master's degree in hand, Charles returned to the corporate headquarters to become vice president for manufacturing.

Charles had learned his caring style of leadership from Bob. During the initial years of the company's development, Bob hired many people in need—some just out of prison, others battling addictions, others just not making it in the world. On top of that, he took them to lunch, gave them motivational books to read, mentored them, and supported them in ways they had never experienced before. Seeing Bob put an emphasis on relationships gave Charles the encouragement to unleash his caring spirit at work. Charles turned whatever job he had at Web into one in which valuing people was at the core. His mission statement, which he wrote a few years before his first neurological symptoms started to appear, shows this passion:

I will make a significant difference in the world by bringing grace with integrity into the lives of others. Therefore, through a disciplined focus, I will apply my life to bringing
  - *peace for people who are in turmoil;*
  - *healing for those who are wounded;*

- *hope for those in despair; and*
- *purpose for those who are drifting.*

Charles recited his mission *out loud* to himself absolutely *every* day. That kept him keenly focused each day on his optimistic goal. And it demonstrated why his work was so important to him. He saw his personal mission as making a difference in each employee's life.

Years later, Charles's friend June Sekera, who was preparing to speak at his memorial service, asked me how Charles had become such a caring person. "What was it about his childhood or other life events that shaped him into this caring man?"

"I'm not sure," I replied. "I guess it was his background as a preacher, when he started preaching as a teenager. I bet he just took that passion for people and brought it into the business environment. But I'll check with Charles's brothers to see if they can shed any light on this."

When I asked Ken, Charles's younger brother, why Charles was such a caring person, Ken replied, "I don't know. He was always that way." After some thought, he added, "As you know, Janet, my parents, with their archaic view of life, didn't have many social skills. As a minister, you'd think that Dad would be able to work a room, but he couldn't. And I never remember my dad giving me a hug or saying 'I love you' until a few years before he died. But Charles filled that void for us. Charles wanted to make everything and everyone okay. When I had a problem, I went to Charles, not my parents. Charles always told me how things would get better.

"One of the times we moved—I must have been about six and Charles was twelve—I remember Dad saying that we couldn't take my tricycle. I was devastated. Then Charles talked to me and said that I was getting bigger and would now be able to ride his bicycle, so I wouldn't need my tricycle anymore. That was all I needed to hear to feel better.

"After Charles went away to college in Florida, I was surprised when Coach Johnson, my high school football coach, relayed to me that Charles had called, 'wondering how Ken was doing.' Mom and Dad never came to one of my games. But whenever Charles was home, he did. My parents never taught us a sense of unity as a family—Charles tried to do that. For as long as I can remember, Charles was always taking care of others."

To fulfill his mission in the face of his disease, Charles now needed that care from others.

Caregiving Affirmation:
Hold on to your passions, because they are
the essence of who you are.

COMMITTED TO HIS "DAILY PERSONAL VICTORY"

Throughout this early stage of the disease, Charles kept his daily commitments and routines. In addition to reciting his mission every morning, he also went on a daily three-mile run.

He'd begun the daily run in 1994. In May, Charles attended a conference at the Mount Washington Hotel in Bretton Woods, New Hampshire. The hotel overlooked the highest peak in New England, which gave the hotel its name—a perfect setting for a seminar targeted at business professionals seeking self-improvement. Inspired, Charles came home committed to jogging every day. "Running every day is not for my health," he insisted. "I made this commitment as my daily personal victory."

The concept of a daily personal victory comes from the teachings of Stephen Covey in his book, *The 7 Habits of Highly Effective People.* Covey suggests that each of us find something that we can do every day to give us a sense of accomplishment and renewal, no matter what else happens. This advice came at just the right time in Charles's life, so he took it to heart. He felt that he was encountering resistance from some senior managers at Web in implementing his progressive concepts of leadership and participative management. That—and probably his recent angioplasty—had him feeling down quite frequently.

In the ten or so years before that conference, Charles had run very little. At one point, while we lived in Atlanta, he barely trained to jog with me in the popular Peachtree Road Race 10K on July 4. Quite a number of years had elapsed since his high school cross-country track days in Searcy, Arkansas. The track team there often won the state championships. Though he wasn't the fastest on the team, running just under a six-minute mile, he was its captain because of his talent for encouraging his teammates. He never felt coordinated enough to participate in other sports, but running came easily to him.

After the conference, Charles told me, "Janet, I've decided that I am going to run every day. I was thinking about starting with one mile and working up to three."

But with my exercise science background, I just had to say, "Starting slow is a good plan, and three miles in the long run should be very doable. But what will you do if you get sick? It's not good to run when you have a fever or a bad cold. Are you sure you need to commit to running *every* day?"

"Yes," he insisted, "I'm going to run every day. It's my way to have a victory every day, no matter what else happens that day." To Charles, missing a day was not even a consideration.

By the time his neurological symptoms appeared, he'd already kept his pledge for a year. He wasn't about to let this new menace get in the way of his commitment, so he kept running, never missing a day, even though his gait became more unstable. Every Tuesday on the calendar in his leather-bound appointment book, he methodically tallied the number of weeks he had run.

Little did Charles know how challenging it would become to keep this promise.

Caregiving Affirmation:
You'll be strengthened by continuing to work
toward your important goals.

AS IF LIFE WERE STILL NORMAL

Our newly renovated kitchen provided the perfect setting for hosting informal dinner parties, something we enjoyed doing to stay connected with our friends. They included Charles's friends from the ESOP community, professors from Boston College's Leadership for Change program, in which Charles served as a business partner, and business colleagues. Typically, Charles prepared pasta with various toppings while everyone gathered and nibbled on snacks. Then we would sit around the dining room table for invigorating discussions. "Let's hope Clinton will be able to . . ." "Did you read that book on leadership by . . . ?" "Did you hear how that company is transforming its employee ownership culture?" "What will happen to the world economy if . . . ?" "What do you think about the principles espoused by . . . ?" Charles stayed passionately involved in every part of each discussion.

We also developed a new weekend ritual. Charles insisted we go to a local sandwich shop at least once to get his favorite sandwich—stir-fried chicken on a submarine roll, with all the veggies, including "hots," but no cheese or sauce. It wasn't easy for him to keep the messy sandwich in one piece and get it to his mouth without spilling half of it, but we didn't miss a weekend.

And we continued other weekend activities that we enjoyed—seeing new movies, walking around town, shopping at the mall, decorating or fixing some new section of our house, eating out at our favorite Indian or Italian restaurants, and attending the occasional musical in Boston. With Charles's symptoms progressing, primarily impacting his movement and vision, it might have made sense for us to reevaluate our lifestyle and priorities. Should we have focused on new missions together? What else should we have done with our lives in light of what we were starting to face? At the time, though, we both continued living life as if all was still normal, both following our passions. Not to have done so would have felt like defeat. We worried about the worst, but we hoped for the best. We didn't talk or think about changing our lifestyle, because we didn't yet realize that we would have to.

Caregiving Affirmation:
Stay focused on what you enjoy.

OUR AUSCHWITZ EXPERIENCE

Charles and I had several times experienced the thrill of overseas travel. A trip in 1990 to Japan, Thailand, and Hong Kong for his executive MBA program at Georgia State University delighted us. In 1993, the nonprofit Shared Participation Foundation in Hungary invited Charles to speak about his management style at its conference in Budapest—and I accompanied him. How exciting to be in a former Communist country—and how beautiful it all was!

Then, at the Bretton Woods conference, Charles met a woman from France whose words would launch us on our next big trip. Charles explained to me that at the conference, a speaker named Joseph Jaworski had shared his childhood experiences. Jaworski's father, Leon, was the famous special prosecutor after the Watergate scandal. When the elder Jaworski was a young lawyer, he had inspected some of the concentration camps after World War II, in preparation for the Nuremberg trials. While working on the trials at home, he told his son Joe not to enter his study under any circumstances. But, as Joe asked the audience, "What is the first thing a young boy does when told not to?" He paused, and then said, "I went into the study." There he saw photographs from the concentration camps, depicting emaciated prisoners and other horrors. Charles told me that Joe sobbed for at least five minutes when telling this story—even though Joe had seen the pictures more than forty years earlier, they still affected him powerfully.

Then a woman in the audience stood up and spoke in French, with her daughter providing an English translation. She shared how her father, a Jew, had been sent to Auschwitz during the war and was killed there. Both Joe's story and hers touched Charles deeply. So when that same woman sent out a mailing to announce a few months later that she was coordinating a trip to Auschwitz, Charles signed us up immediately.

The trip was to include visits to the concentration camps in the morning, then lectures and discussions in the afternoons and evenings, which sounded easy enough to handle. However, by the time the trip finally arrived about a year later, the disease had more forcefully affected Charles's vision and movements. Climbing down stairs continued to give him his greatest difficulty, and, as we soon learned, getting up and down from the floor was very hard for him. At this point Charles was not yet ready to accept any assistance from others—even me. He was fiercely independent. But wouldn't you know it! The meeting room for this conference was on the second floor, and there was no elevator. And eating was often outside—sitting on the stairs or the ground. I can still remember Charles holding his tray of food while maneuvering down the stairs to find a place to sit. His food nearly slid off the tray a number of times, but somehow he managed to hide his disease from everyone. He even continued to jog every day along the streets of Poland.

Despite the physical hardships for Charles, this adventure enriched our lives and our world understanding. The most powerful experience of the trip for Charles was in the original brick buildings at the heart of the camp. Thousands of mug shots of newly arrived prisoners covered every inch of the inside walls. I, too, felt awe at the sheer number of pictures, each representing one prisoner—one unique person. But Charles looked deeply into the faces peering out of the pictures. He seemed to be able to see into the heart of each person, feeling their fear of just having arrived at the camp, being separated from loved ones, stripped of all their clothes and belongings, having their head shaved, and dressing in the striped clothing of prisoners. It was as if Charles related to each individual emotionally. Later, whenever we would show friends pictures from that trip, Charles would say that from those prisoners' perspective, life was very precious. That was Charles's gift—seeing the inner needs and concerns of each person. The experience forced both of us, through the pain of understanding the atrocities at Auschwitz, to learn and grow.

Charles would soon face his own Auschwitz as his body deteriorated, leaving him a prisoner within it.

Caregiving Affirmation:
Feel all of life's emotions.

2

※

1996: The Delicate Balance
of Working Together

ACCOMMODATING THE MOUNTING CHANGES

Not even a full year into this disease and our daily routine was already changing.

Each morning, after a restless night of not sleeping well, Charles prepared for his day. He was still able to step over the high rim of the tub and shower on his own without incident. He continued to dress himself, with a few struggles. His fingers would defy him when he'd try to button his shirtsleeves. Though he was reluctant for me to do so, I began to take on that task. And then he'd get frustrated trying to knot his silk tie. As he lost the coordination to loop its ends around, I stepped in. At first that created a problem for me, as I didn't know how to tie a man's tie. And then once I learned, he was rarely happy with the off-kilter knot I made.

Before leaving the bedroom, Charles would down his new designer pills touted as having superantioxidants powerful enough to preserve brain health. He'd become a guinea pig because scientists hadn't—and still haven't—found a cure, or even an effective treatment for the diseases they hypothesized he might have. We hoped to discover, by trial and error, something that would stop the disease's relentless progression.

Once Charles was dressed and ready, the stairs were his next obstacle. With our bedroom on the second floor and our house sitting on a hill, Charles had to maneuver down more than two flights of stairs. He would carefully lower each foot to reach the next step, his deteriorating depth perception compromising his navigating ability. To provide additional support for Charles, we'd recently installed handrails on the elegant front stairway inside our hundred-year-old Victorian home.

Charles still drove the twenty miles or so to the small corporate headquarters where he worked, but I insisted he take the old silver Dodge Aries I had bought from my grandmother's estate after she died in 1989. The new champagne-colored Ford Taurus needed better care than he could usually provide, his carelessness with food and drinks in the car now worsened by his diminished control over his body.

At work, Charles's difficulties persisted. His typical duties as vice president of manufacturing included attending meetings, conducting phone conversations, reading reports, working on projects, and developing strategic plans. Each day's tasks invariably required reading. His eyes struggled to track across the page, making it difficult to get from line to line. At times this was compounded by double vision—his eyes were not working well together. And because he also had difficulty seeing and recognizing objects, he moved his most-used file folders into an open holder on the wide windowsill next to his desk.

Soon his beautiful, distinctive writing style began to deteriorate into squiggly lines he could barely control. This made him more dependent on the computer, even though he had never learned to type with more than one finger.

When he arrived home, he would still chop and grill and stir, fixing a wonderfully fresh meal we'd eat in our newly renovated kitchen. I've never been a good cook. In fact, I hate to cook, so Charles had taken on this task for us. Watching him now, I wondered, *How much longer will he be able to wield a knife and handle the utensils required for cooking? And what will we do if I have to start doing the cooking?* Those thoughts, however, took a backseat to my worry about how Charles would feel when he lost this ability.

On a typical evening, we would simply watch the news on a major TV network and then one of our favorite sitcoms, such as *Mad About You* or *Frasier.* Finally, we would prepare for an early bedtime.

During our evening conversation, Charles often complained, "I just feel spacey all day. I don't feel like myself."

"Maybe it's those experimental drugs you're taking," I'd respond, not really knowing if the culprit was the drugs or the advancing disease. And I could tell that even with the new sleeping pills and antidepressants he was taking, his bouts of insomnia and depression were growing more frequent.

"My feet don't feel like my own," Charles would also say. "I look at them, and cognitively, I know they're mine, but they don't *feel* like mine."

When we had asked Dr. Ravin, his neurologist, about this strangest symptom yet, she had replied, "When your limbs feel detached from your body, it's called *alien limb phenomenon.*"

"Are you feeling that funny sensation tonight?" I asked him.

"Yes," he answered, "and it's such a weird feeling."

How could all of these losses have happened within just the first year that this disease had become evident? Somehow, Charles and I resiliently adjusted our daily tasks to accommodate his internal thief.

Caregiving Affirmation:
You can handle losses if you take them as they come.

I BLEW IT

I didn't realize how sensitive Charles was about whether or not to tell others about his condition until the day I blew it.

When his first symptoms started to develop, he mentioned that he didn't want to tell anyone—not his friends, not his work colleagues, and not even our families. "I'm afraid they'll fire me if they find out," he said, not wanting to lose the job he loved.

"What about talking to Carolyn?" I asked, referring to my sister, who is trained in speech therapy. "Don't you think she would be helpful now?"

Charles agreed that we could confide in her. When she had lived in Arizona, Carolyn had worked with people who had Parkinson's disease. Midway through her wedding reception, about ten of her patients sat in chairs placed in a semicircle. Carolyn sat in the center, her puffy white wedding gown flowing to the floor. We all looked on with astonishment as she led them in songs like "Hey, Look Me

Over." Though many of the patients had difficulty speaking, all could sing.

I thought that Carolyn's experience with neurological diseases might help Charles at this point, as his speech had already started to slow. Charles agreed, giving the okay to tell her. But though Carolyn encouraged him to tell others, he continued to refuse. Charles wanted to keep his condition very private. He thought he could hide it.

I, on the other hand, had difficulty keeping this tragedy to myself. My way of coping at this stage was to talk about it with family and dear friends; I had found relief and support by sharing the news with a few of those people closest to me. And I didn't feel that his fears about getting fired were legitimate. Surely the executive team at Web Industries would not take such extreme measures, and would be supportive. I couldn't convince Charles of this, however; his fear was very real.

I soon found that I couldn't keep it in any longer—I had to tell others about what Charles and I were going through.

I remember the day I told my team at work. At one of our weekly staff meetings, we sat at a table over lunch at a wonderful nearby cafeteria. I was eating the half-portion of the pasta of the day that I usually ordered, and my favorite low-fat chocolate yogurt cake.

Charles and I had been immersed in our research on PSP and CBGD, two of the possible diagnoses. That was how we had learned that both conditions had dismal prognoses. The harsh reality—that Charles actually had a devastating disease—had just become real to me. The fact that he would die young shot straight through my heart.

While I was conducting the staff meeting, my emotions suddenly welled up and overwhelmed me. I needed to tell my team members *something;* I couldn't just continue to talk about the items on our agenda. Giving in to tears, I looked around the table and said, "I need to tell you something. Charles has a neurological disease . . . and the prognosis is not good. It will probably take his life early—maybe in five to ten years."

Everyone expressed sympathy and asked questions to clarify what we knew about the disease, but they really didn't know what to say to this shocking news. As I thought back on it afterward, I wondered if I should have told them. All I knew at the time was that I simply couldn't bear the sadness by myself any longer.

When I told Charles that I had talked to my staff about his illness, he unleashed an anger I had rarely witnessed in him. I don't ever remember his being disappointed with me to the extent that he was over this issue. Such a strong reaction was out of character for him. I could count on one hand the number of fights we had had in our long marriage. I felt hurt; he felt betrayed.

"Who else have you told?" he demanded. I confessed that I had also talked to my close friend Jean and to my family. I felt pangs of guilt that I had broken the trust between us. I worked hard to understand the diverse ways Charles and I handled this issue. I obtained tremendous insight when I participated in the Myers-Briggs inventory training at work.

The Myers-Briggs Type Indicator (MBTI) explores people's preferences on four scales. The "energizing" scale looks at where we like to focus our attention or where we get our energy from, whether outside of us (which is labeled as *extrovert*) or within us (*introvert*). This is a bit different than the way many of us define *extrovert* and *introvert*. The "perceiving" scale shows the way we like to look at things, either focusing on the concrete or on what might be. The "deciding" scale measures whether we typically make our decisions either in a logical way or more from our values. And the "living" scale shows how we deal with the world around us—living a planned and organized life, or living more spontaneously.

I learned when I took the MBTI that I was predominantly extroverted on the "energizing" scale. When he had taken the MBTI a number of years earlier during his executive MBA program, Charles had scored as an introvert. We were opposites when it came to where we got our energy. I got my energy from others; Charles got his from within.

I would have initially guessed that Charles was an extrovert, because he was such a people person. He engaged in intense conversations with others. But as I think more deeply about those conversations, he was always the one asking the questions, finding out a lot about others but revealing little about himself. For Charles, who grew up in a fundamentalist, conservative Christian household, family matters always stayed at home.

During the MBTI program at my job, the company trainer led us in a variety of exercises designed to help participants see the differences on each of the MBTI scales. She also promoted the positive nature of working with this diversity.

The trainer described a scene from the movie *Ordinary People* to help explain the differences between introverts and extroverts. In the movie, Calvin and Beth were Conrad's parents. Conrad had tried to commit suicide after the tragic sailing death of his older brother, and then had been taken to a mental hospital. Recently released, he was back in school but still receiving counseling from a psychiatrist.

When Beth and Calvin were at a birthday party, Beth overheard Calvin telling one of their good friends that Conrad was doing better and was in therapy. On the way home from the party, Beth boiled silently. She finally accused Calvin of going too far in telling all to their friend. She repeated a number of times that this was a "private matter"—just between them—and not to be shared outside of the home.

The trainer described Beth as being an introvert who needed privacy, and Calvin as being an extrovert who found energy, and therefore comfort, in sharing his difficulties with others. I finally understood the tension between Charles and me. As an extrovert, I needed to talk to others to survive. But as an introvert, Charles needed to deal with his issues quietly, within himself.

With this newfound awareness, Charles and I could finally understand our differences.

No matter how wise we are, working through differences like these will always require extra effort. I had to handle not only my sadness at Charles's disease, but also the impact of the different ways that we each dealt with it. And not just with this incident, but with many others throughout the course of the disease. I've learned that couples need to understand these differences in order to discover the delicate balance of working together, which flows out of respect for each other. Through that respect, couples can find the grace and forgiveness they need to overcome conflicts.

Caregiving Affirmation:
When you respect each other's differences,
you can overcome conflicts.

CURIOSITY VERSUS DIGNITY

What could this disease be? Charles's symptoms brought out the scientist in me. As insensitive as this may sound, solving the mystery of his disease almost bordered on being fun for me. Sometimes I would be totally unaware of how my inquisitiveness might be affecting him. Although the physical manifestations of the disease fascinated me, they totally frustrated and embarrassed him.

FIND THE SUGAR PACKET

"Charles, can you find the sugar packet I just put on the table?" I asked as we ate dinner at TGI Friday's, one of our favorite restaurants in Boston. Charles looked down at the table, and I watched his eyes wander around for more than a few seconds. "There," he finally said, pointing to the sugar packet. His peripheral vision didn't kick in right away, like mine would have, allowing me to see it immediately.

Caught up in the intriguing nature of this, I asked, "Charles, can you close your eyes while I hide it again?" Obediently, he closed his eyes, and I moved the sugar packet to another place on the table. "You can open your eyes now. Can you find the sugar packet?" I inquired. And again, it took him a few seconds to see it. It was amazing to me that Charles struggled with something so automatic for most people.

Unfortunately, though, I didn't know when to quit. I kept asking him to close his eyes and then find the sugar packet. Finally, embarrassed and frustrated, Charles refused to play along, saying, "No, Janet. Stop it!" I hadn't paused to think about what it would feel like to be the subject of my experiments.

ANOTHER GAME

Just before Christmas, Charles had an appointment with a neurologist at Boston Medical Center. The doctor spent over an hour examining him, conducting a battery of visual tests that fascinated me. For one, he asked, "Charles, can you draw a clock on this piece of paper?" That required Charles to draw a circle and then place the numbers correctly inside the clock. As I watched, Charles struggled to make the round circle for the outside of the clock. As he maneuvered the pen, he successfully made the appropriate curve on the right side of the clock, but then flattened it as he drew the left side of the circle. And when placing the numbers inside the clock, he couldn't get all of them in their right places, especially the 7, 8, 9, 10, and 11 on the left side of the clock.

When we visited my family in Florida during the holiday, I wanted to show them this new peculiarity. *Maybe it will help them understand the extent of Charles's disease,* I thought. With my entire family sitting around the table after dinner one evening, I got a piece of paper and pencil and asked Charles to draw a clock.

While I found it fascinating to see how the disease had affected Charles's brain—and therefore, his vision—it made Charles feel like a spectacle. He drew the clock, the same way he'd done it in the doctor's office, but then lashed out at me for what he perceived as making fun of him in public: "You're embarrassing me, Janet!" Mortified, he clammed up and wouldn't say another word or even look at me. And my family, looking on, didn't know what to say, either, uncomfortable at being a part of this encounter.

It wasn't until after Charles died that I really admitted I had probably gone too far in my morbid curiosity. I shared the sugar-packet story with some of my commuter friends on the train while traveling home from Boston. When I finished, one of them, a licensed social worker, just came out with it, saying, "That's mean!" In retrospect, I acknowledged that she was right. Even though I hadn't intended to be insensitive, I was.

At the time, I didn't fully realize just how much Charles still wanted to hide any weakness or vulnerability. He wanted everyone to think he was still normal, and, more important, *he* still wanted to *believe* that he was normal. I had no bad intentions; I just continued to have a hard time judging when my fascination took Charles out of his comfort zone. Our approaches to this disease had clashed again.

NOSE PROBLEMS

At one point, Charles insisted that I pluck his nose hairs. They were bothering him, he said, and he thought the only solution was to pluck them. *Yuck.* I found the thought of doing that too gross. I was happy to do many other things for him, but not pluck nose hairs.

Charles continued to insist, so for my own sanity, I decided that I had to at least try. Gingerly reaching in with tweezers, I plucked only a few hairs close to the front. But to Charles, that wasn't enough. Every night, he would insist that I pluck more nose hairs.

It wasn't until my mother visited that we discovered the source of Charles's irritation. "Maybe it is just some hardened mucus inside his nose," she suggested. "Why don't you rub a little of my Blistex up into his nasal passage," she added, handing me the tube that would rescue me from my dreaded task. Charles quickly felt relief, and we recognized that it wasn't the nose hairs causing him the irritation, but instead, the dryness. I became his official nose cleaner.

Thinking back on this incident, I wondered why I hadn't thought of the cause of the problem and an appropriate solution on my own. Why hadn't it dawned on me that because he had lost much of the motor control in his hands, he hadn't been able to blow or clean out his own nose? I had thought that Charles's insistence on my plucking his nose hairs was just another one of those curious aspects of this disease.

Caregiving Affirmation:
Use empathy to preserve your loved one's dignity.

STILL TRAVELING—AND STILL HIDING HIS DISEASE

ADVENTURES TO THE BRITISH ISLES

At this point, Charles still had no intention of slowing down. The disease gradually inched its way through his brain, but no one besides us was allowed to know. This became difficult, however, when we traveled to London.

Todd, a former Web Industries employee, was serving with his family as a missionary in a suburb of London. Todd had given us a standing invitation to visit anytime, so when an employee ownership group in Scotland requested that Charles speak at its conference, we decided that we would visit Todd and his family in London together, and then Charles would travel on his own from there to Scotland.

We weren't going to miss this opportunity. About a year earlier, before any signs of this disease had appeared, the same group had invited Charles to speak at their conference, but they weren't able to fund his trip. At the time, I was between jobs and uncomfortable with our financial situation. "I don't think we should take the chance of going until I have a job offer," I said, reluctantly convincing Charles not to go.

Charles had always regretted that decision. He felt he had missed a significant chance to spread his passion for employee ownership and to enjoy the special thrill of traveling abroad. And I felt bad that I had caused him to miss that opportunity. I vowed to myself not to be an obstacle in the future. Chances like those are precious and should not be passed up, so in January of 1996, he accepted this most recent invitation, and we took the trip across the pond.

Because Charles still refused to tell others about his developing neurological disease, the normal challenges of travel were compounded: We had to try to hide his condition. The first test came in maneuvering around the typically tiny London flat that Todd, his wife Donna, and their children lived in. It was just one room wide, with the living room and kitchen occupying the first floor and all the bedrooms taking up the second. To get to the only bathroom, also on the second floor, we had to climb a narrow, steep staircase.

Luckily, the first-floor living room was converted into our guest bedroom with the use of a pull-out couch. However, we still had to use the bathroom on the second floor. Charles couldn't navigate these stairs on his own—especially coming down—so I tried to nonchalantly assist him. We did our best to hide Charles's condition, but Todd and Donna both commented later, once Charles's disease was out in the open, that they had noticed the problem. They were kind enough not to embarrass Charles by asking about it during our visit.

As Charles and I toured London, mostly on our own, Charles did quite well. I held his arm as we maneuvered through the crowds. "They appear to be floating . . . and they are doing it so gracefully," Charles said once as people walked by. This was another curious manifestation of how the neurological damage affected the movement of his eyes.

We took the London subway frequently to travel around the city. As the subway train pulled into a station and was coming to a stop, a taped announcement blared, "Mind the gap!" It didn't take long for us to understand what that meant. But it still provided another challenge for Charles as he carefully stepped in and out of the train over the gaping space between subway car and platform—not an easy task with people pushing from behind.

After we had a lovely visit in London—seeing Big Ben, the parliament in session, Westminster Abbey, and Buckingham Palace—I reluctantly flew home to go back to work. I wondered if Charles was nervous about not having my assistance for the rest of his trip. He then traveled alone north to Glasgow. When making the arrangements for the trip, the CEO of his company had encouraged Charles to take the train from England to Scotland instead of flying. "You'll enjoy the wonderful countryside," the CEO had said, marveling at its beauty.

But the train ride, on top of the rest of the trip, totally exhausted Charles physically. We didn't realize just how much, though, until his first day back at work after he'd returned from Scotland. I got a call at work late that morning from Sharon in Charles's office. "Janet, I don't mean to alarm you," she said in her soft, sweet voice, "but Charles collapsed here at work. We called the ambulance, and they've taken him to University of Massachusetts Medical Center." Even though the people in Charles's office didn't know about his neurological condition, they were well aware of his former heart problems, which caused them concern.

"What happened?" I asked.

She responded, "He was in his office talking to Al when his eyes rolled to the back of his head and he just collapsed. He hit his head on the edge of the desk when he slumped to the floor. He got a pretty bad gash."

"I'll get to the hospital as fast as I can," I said.

My drive there took forty-five minutes. On the way, I panicked, thinking about the possibilities. Was this related to his heart, or was it a seizure caused by the neurological condition? Either way, I still felt I couldn't mention his disease to his colleagues.

When I arrived at the hospital, I found Charles in the emergency room, with his friends from work. Charles was doing better, albeit with a few stitches in his head. He was alert and smiling, and mostly seemed embarrassed about the whole event.

After monitoring Charles's heart, the doctor confirmed that he hadn't had a recurrence of his heart problem. "His collapse was most likely caused by exhaustion from his trip," he added. "Go home and get some rest," he prescribed.

You can imagine my total exasperation that evening when Charles, determined not to miss even one day of running, went out for his daily jog. I couldn't stop him no matter how persuasively I argued. How I sighed in relief when he walked in the door later, having made it back home safely!

Charles continued to vehemently resist accepting the deterioration already beginning in his body. Unfortunately, this denial would endanger him in the coming years.

SCARES IN CHINA

That May, Charles and I capitalized on another once-in-a-lifetime opportunity. The National Center for Employee Ownership (NCEO) in the United States was coordinating its second annual conference on enterprise reform and market opportunities with a corresponding group in Beijing. The NCEO invited Charles to speak about employee ownership at Web Industries.

I didn't want to miss out on this experience—and Charles needed my support physically.

Just prior to our trip, relations between China and the United States had begun to crumble. U.S. businesses were complaining about the Chinese government's lack of control over the rampant pirating of copyrighted materials, such as music CDs and books. The Chinese saw this copying as a form of flattery. They've been copying their own artists and masters for thousands of years. Because of the tensions, though, a number of Chinese businesspeople who were already registered for the conference canceled at the last minute. Nevertheless, the conference continued, though attendance was lower than in the previous year.

After speaking on the first day of the conference, Charles told me about his disappointment. "I didn't do very well. I don't think I con-nected with this group like I have with others." I wondered if this perception was fueled by how the disease was slowing his speech and possibly affecting his presentation abilities, such as gestures and facial expressions. Nonetheless, his American colleagues assured him that he had done well.

The resulting stress, however, must have affected him physically. That evening in our hotel room, his chest pain returned. Charles hadn't experienced chest pain in quite some time. Fortunately, we still carried his nitroglycerin; putting one pill under his tongue did the trick. The pain subsided. But this nerve-racking experience put me on edge for the rest of the trip.

Once the three-day conference had ended, Charles and I, along with some of the other American speakers and conference coordinators, toured Beijing and the surrounding area. Charles did fine walking everywhere. His only major challenge came when we climbed the Great Wall of China, with its thousands of steps.

For the climb, my assistance didn't provide enough support for Charles. We asked Julie, the conference planner from the NCEO, to help. Because Charles was still adamantly opposed to telling people about his neurological condition, he told her he was having some vision problems. Without any questions, Julie grabbed one of Charles's arms, and I took the other. We climbed step by step, passing the many vendors crowding the way, until we reached the top of that section of wall. From there, we could view miles of the Chinese landscape sprinkled with ancient portions of the Great Wall. What a memorable sight!

During the trip, we also toured Tian'anmen Square, the former Imperial Palace in the Forbidden City, the largest shrine in China called the Temple of Heaven, and the Summer Palace for former emperors. Occasionally some Chinese families would stop me and ask if they could take my picture. Apparently, some of the people from the countryside who were visiting Beijing had not seen many blondes before. We found watching the Chinese going about their everyday lives most interesting—getting haircuts on the sidewalk, snacking on fried chicken feet (eating bones and all!), playing with live chicks in the park, doing tai chi, competing with each other at board games along the sidewalk, and riding their bicycles—in mass numbers—everywhere they went.

Then, on our flight home, we had another scare.

We hadn't experienced any problems on our thirteen-hour-plus trip to China. Charles and I had had a nice chat with the woman sitting next to us. She had traveled to China many times and gave us suggestions about places to visit. We'd been delighted to discover that she would be on the flight home with us, as well. Charles and I had taken sleeping pills on the trip over to China in hopes of fighting jet lag when we arrived. We took the prescription-only drug Ambien, which I had obtained from one of our doctors. Just after the flight attendants brought our dinner, Charles and I each took a pill. Before we knew it, we were landing in Beijing.

On the way home, we tried the same approach. I gave Charles his sleeping pill again after our first meal. But then we remembered that the woman we had met on our flight over should be on this plane, too. She had told us that she would be sitting in the second-floor section of the 747, so with difficulty, I assisted Charles up the winding, narrow stairs to the second level, where we found our new friend. After talking with her for a while, Charles appeared to pass out while still standing. We rushed to sit him in someone's seat and called the flight attendant.

My heart plunged as I immediately thought of the worst-case scenario: *Is he having a heart attack?* This fear felt real to me because of the chest-pain incident in the hotel. "Charles, Charles," I said as I shook his arm. I tried one more time. "Charles!" Nothing aroused him. After surveying the situation, the flight attendant retrieved her medical bag. She took his pulse and blood pressure. "They are fine," she said. "But because of your husband's past heart condition, the pilot wants to land in Anchorage, Alaska, to get him medical help." Landing in Alaska—would that be necessary? Would we be whisked off to a hospital there? *Yikes.*

Sitting next to Charles in someone else's seat, I began to relax enough to realize the source of the problem. I had given Charles the Ambien before we'd made our trek up the stairs. The pill must have kicked in more quickly than we'd expected, and Charles had just fallen sound asleep.

After about forty-five minutes, he finally started to awaken a bit. Though it wasn't easy to do so, I finally convinced the flight attendant of the likelihood of my sleeping-pill theory, and that it wouldn't be necessary for the pilot to land the plane in Alaska. Once Charles was more awake, some people helped me move him back down the stairs and to our seats, where we finished the rest of the journey without further incident.

In spite of all the scares, that trip afforded us many precious memories, and was an experience I would gladly repeat.

TACKLING THE OLYMPICS

Atlanta knew how to get the Olympic Committee's attention. In 1989, just before we had moved from Atlanta to Boston, I pounded the hot pavement, jogging with thousands of others through the downtown streets of Atlanta. The city of Atlanta organized the road race to demonstrate to the Olympic Committee its skill in coordinating this type of event. When the committee announced that Atlanta had won the bid for hosting the 1996 Olympics, Charles and I looked forward to visiting one of our favorite places, and to attending this world event.

I signed up for as many events as possible. Because of the random drawing for seats, we received tickets for only a few days' worth of track and field events, and for team handball. But that was good enough for us.

Since our move from Atlanta, my brother Doug had relocated to a suburb there. That made it easy for our visit—except that all the bedrooms in his house were on the second floor. Charles and I struggled each day, again trying to mask the difficulty he faced with each step.

Doug had planned in advance to get us into the Olympic spirit. Our first day out, Charles wore a black polo shirt with a red collar and the Olympic insignia, which Doug had bought for him. It looked fabulous with his dark, graying hair and his trim body, thinner now than when we'd lived in Atlanta. I dressed in a red, white, and blue polo shirt that Doug had given me, along with a wide-brimmed straw hat with a red, white, and blue ribbon encircling the lower portion.

As we entered the new Olympic Stadium with thousands of other spectators for the track and field events, the aroma of popcorn and hot dogs permeated the warm Atlanta air. But then our formidable nemesis appeared yet again—the stadium stairs! Doug's staircase paled in comparison. The shorter but wider stadium steps made walking up tricky for Charles. If we had needed to climb them only once, that would have been okay. But each time Charles needed to use the restroom, we had to tackle them again.

We decided to pass on going to the team handball event, and instead gave our tickets to my sister Sue and her daughter, who were also visiting. The bombing at the Olympic Park in downtown Atlanta occurred just before we arrived. So on top of having to keep Charles steady, I was anxious, hoping that no other terrorist events would occur during our walk around the shops, park, and restaurants.

What an opportunity—attending the Olympics! But from my perspective, Charles's feat in climbing the stadium stairs beat the performances of all the athletes tossing hammers, racing toward the finish line, or jumping with poles.

Caregiving Affirmation:
Explore life's adventures together to store up
fond memories that will sustain you.

TREATMENTS PROVIDE A SENSE OF CONTROL

SAYING "AH"

Many neurological diseases affect speech. In this early stage of Charles's disease, his speech first slowed, then became softer. Still fighting to maintain his optimistic attitude, he commented, "I always tended to speak too quickly most of the time, so my slower speech is probably a good thing."

My sister Carolyn, the speech therapist, instructed Charles in a variety of exercises to help him maintain his voice's volume and his articulation.

The first exercise she gave him was to practice saying *ah*. She instructed him to say it as loudly as he could, and to hold it for as long as possible. Carolyn said that people with neurological diseases hear themselves at a loud volume, but actually speak more quietly than they think they are. She explained the importance of strengthening the vocal cords by holding the *ah's*. When Charles first tried this exercise, it surprised me that he couldn't project well and that his voice petered out so quickly. Because he practiced every day, though, he improved his volume. At one point, he actually started to speak too loudly. It took a while for him to learn to adjust his volume to the appropriate level.

Carolyn gave us many other exercises, most of which Charles didn't continue practicing. But the one, in addition to the *ah's*, that we stuck with was a word exercise. I gave Charles a word or phrase, and he put it into a sentence. This became fun and challenging for him.

At times, he would get frustrated that he couldn't do these exercises as well as he had hoped. Nonetheless, they gave him a sense of control. They helped him to focus on a more positive outlook—that he *could* do something to stem the progression of this disease, and to feel he was not just a victim.

Caregiving Affirmation:
Actively work to minimize the feeling of being a victim.

A STRING OF BEADS

Dr. Hammer was a nonstop talker. Once Charles got back in the exam room where there were all types of gadgets, his appointments with this optometrist lasted over an hour. Dr. Hammer, a maverick in vision care, expressed his disappointment with many ophthalmologists who don't give hope to their patients. He believed that eye exercises could improve the vision of people with neurological conditions. He was determined to give it a try with Charles, and Charles was as a willing patient.

Before seeing Dr. Hammer, Charles had begun having trouble reading. He'd lost his ability to track his eyes across a line of text on a page or a computer screen, and then get to the next line. Losing his visual capabilities, especially reading, became his next greatest fear after the fear of losing his speech.

Charles had, as he would say, "ten thousand books." And I believed him, having moved boxes and boxes of them every time we bought a new house. He called books his friends. He loved to read. He shared this passion by buying multiple copies of his favorite books and giving them away to his friends and colleagues.

After his first appointment with Dr. Hammer, Charles came home with a brown bag full of stuff. I wasn't sure that Charles could even remember how to use it all. I figured I would need to go to the next appointment with him to learn the exercise routines and ensure that he practiced them correctly.

The exercise that seemed to hold the best hope for helping him involved using four different-colored beads that were strung at about six-inch intervals. Charles held one end of the string at his nose and the other end as far out as his other arm could reach. Dr. Hammer had instructed Charles to look at the closest bead, then the next, and on down the line until he got to the last bead, and then to go back to the first.

Another exercise had Charles looking at a picture on the wall— the watercolor painting from Budapest that we had hanging in our bedroom. Charles said, "Dr. Hammer told me to look at one corner, then the next. After I finish looking at each corner, I'm supposed to look at the middle of the picture." We placed small sticky notes on each corner and in the middle of our painting to help facilitate this exercise.

The simplest exercise, yet one that was still very difficult for Charles, was to look close, then far. He held his thumb up by his nose and would focus on it for a few seconds. Then he would look at an object farther way. He finished by returning his gaze back to his thumb.

In addition to assigning the exercises, Dr. Hammer ordered various pairs of glasses for Charles, who had never worn any before. Ultimately, I'm not sure that the exercises or the glasses really helped; but for the short term, they gave him hope that he could have some measure of control over potential losses.

Eventually, the time commitment required to perform all the exercises and visit Dr. Hammer became too burdensome. Not only did Dr. Hammer talk a lot, but the drive to and from his office was about forty-five minutes each way. Though he stuck with wearing the glasses, Charles eventually abandoned the hope that the exercises and the visits had initially inspired.

DRUGS KEEP FAILING

There were always new drug regimens to try, because the old drugs kept seeming to fail.

One of the first drugs that Dr. Ravin prescribed for Charles was

Eldepryl. Apparently, it is a superpowerful antioxidant. She told us that some early studies showed that this drug might help slow down the degeneration caused by neurological diseases. Parlodel, which Dr. Ravin also gave to Charles at this time, was supposed to help in a similar way. About the same time that Charles started taking these two drugs, he also began taking Elavil for his persistent insomnia. One of these drugs, or a combination of them, made Charles feel spacey. Regardless of whether they would help him in the long run, he insisted, "I don't want to feel like this all the time." So he refused to continue taking them.

Then Dr. Ravin gave him amantadine syrup. Sometimes the syrup relieves the fatigue associated with Parkinson's symptoms, though scientists aren't sure why it does. Dr. Ravin might have figured that it would help Charles because Parkinson's is a neurodegenerative disease, just as Charles's disease was. But one Sunday morning after Charles and I got our favorite bagels—mine with a cinnamon glazed, and his a cinnamon raisin—he started complaining. "I feel weird," he said.

"Can you describe what you mean a little better to me?" I asked.

"I just feel weird," was all he would say.

When this happened consistently for a few weeks after we got bagels, Charles began to think that the bagels caused the weird feeling. But Charles and I had been eating bagels for years, so they couldn't have been the culprit. We finally decided that amantadine could possibly be the cause. Charles didn't measure out the serving of the liquid medication, so he may have been taking too much with each dose. Because we hadn't noticed any lessening of his symptoms since he'd been taking it, Charles stopped taking it.

I'm sure Dr. Ravin wasn't pleased that Charles just discontinued taking medications that he didn't like without consulting her first. But we did tell her after the fact on subsequent visits.

Each time a drug or therapy didn't succeed in helping Charles, his frustration and disappointment intensified. How was he supposed to stop the barreling progression of this condition when the side effects from the drugs were worse than the symptoms?

Caregiving Affirmation:
Treatments won't always work. This isn't *your* failure.

STILL RUNNING DESPITE NASTY FALLS

Charles's running commitment afforded him a feeling of control while other losses started to creep in. And it was truly amazing to watch him run so gracefully while other movements were becoming more difficult. He faithfully went out every day for his three-mile run, which served as his daily personal victory.

But this was not without risk.

Charles usually ran in the mornings. But one morning he'd missed the opportunity, so he ran later that evening—after dark. I had already prepared myself for bed and was watching TV when Charles entered the bedroom after his run. I didn't notice the skinned knee and elbow—because my eyes were focused on the blood dripping down his entire face.

"I just tripped on something in the road," Charles said, minimizing the situation when he saw the panic on my face.

"How far out were you when it happened?" I asked.

"About a mile or so down Commonwealth Avenue," he replied.

"Oh no! You had to run all the way back like that?" I exclaimed.

When I figured out that he really was okay, I couldn't resist grabbing the camera sitting on the desk. Charles chuckled as I took his picture—but even though this seems odd, I just had to document the grotesqueness of his blood-drenched face.

Then I quickly provided first aid, carefully washing the fresh wounds on his face. As I cleaned him up, the line of horrid abrasions came into full view. They went from his forehead down to his nose, cheek, and chin.

We later scouted the area where he thought he had fallen, and we noticed a large tree root system growing into the street. That must have been what brought him down. However, when most of us trip and fall, we catch ourselves with our hands. Or, if we do it correctly, we drop and roll. But Charles, with this neurological condition, couldn't do either. When he tripped, he plunged straight onto his face.

I tried to use this fall to warn Charles about the progression of the disease—and the fact that he needed to be very careful. But he refused to accept that the disease had anything to do with his fall. He insisted that he'd just tripped because it was dark. Though it was dark and he'd most likely tripped, I still believed that falling flat on his face was a by-product of the disease's damage. I worried that his denial and lack of concern about safety would put him at greater risk for more falls—or possibly, something even worse.

But Charles's attitude preserved his belief that running was still within his scope of control. Throughout the disease's progression, he stuck to his running commitment with determination. It kept him from feeling handicapped.

After that fall, I tried to run with him most of the time, hoping that I would be able to catch him if he tripped. Luckily for me, the disease had started to slow down his running, allowing me to keep up with him despite my slower pace. That autumn, however, held several nasty spills for him.

The next tumble came a few months later while I jogged with him. We ran on the sidewalks of our neighborhood in Newton, Massachusetts, a small city founded in the 1600s. Unfortunately, many of Newton's old cement sidewalks were cracked, tilted up or down on one side or another, or had missing pieces. Even the smallest deformities in these sidewalks posed a threat to Charles. About one mile into this particular Saturday-morning run, Charles tripped and fell. My hope of catching him had been in vain. How quickly someone goes down when he trips! Again, he stumbled directly onto his face, scraping similar areas as in that first terrible fall. Blood started to ooze from the fresh wounds.

A man carrying a carton of bagels happened to walk by just as Charles fell. He stopped immediately and asked, "Can I help? I work right here. Why don't you come in, and we'll clean you up and make sure you're okay."

Charles quickly replied in embarrassment, "I'm fine; we'll just run on home." But home was more than a mile away.

"Charles, let's go in and make sure you are okay; then we'll see about getting home," I pleaded. Charles reluctantly agreed.

When we arrived in the office, we learned that the man was a dentist. In the midst of patients coming for their appointments and meeting with the hygienists, this dentist and his staff brought us the supplies we needed to help clean Charles's abrasions.

Once Charles was fairly well cleaned up, the dentist asked, "Can I drive you home?" I immediately said yes, while Charles kept insisting that he could make it home on foot. Finally, though, the dentist talked Charles into letting him drive us home.

In reflecting on the dentist's kindness, Charles often remarked, "This disease brings out the best in people. That dentist left a busy office with patients and drove me home. Can you believe that?"

"Yeah," I agreed. "Your disease allows others to give. That makes *them* feel good as well."

Charles continued to struggle with his own acceptance of his condition and what that might mean for his running. But the support from strangers helped remind him of the goodness of human nature, a wonderful consequence of his personal tragedy.

Caregiving Affirmation:
Your loved one's struggles can bring out
the best in you and in others.

His Biggest Loss to Date

I had noticed for some time Charles's increasing anxiety while driving. He continued to hug the lane line to the left and seemed quite uptight, grasping the steering wheel hard. But whenever I said something to him, he denied having a problem driving. He always brought up his experience of driving a truck to deliver the *Tampa Tribune* while in college. "I was a professional driver," he'd retort.

Now in the early stages of this disease, he'd already had a few minor accidents resulting in bumps and dents on the car. One happened while he drove down the Southeast Expressway in Boston with its three cramped, always-busy lanes of traffic. "A truck moved out of its lane and brushed my car," he said, totally believing that the incident was the truck driver's fault. I'm sure, though, that Charles had drifted into the truck's lane.

It was clear to me that he had to stop driving. But then what would we do?

I worked in Boston, and he worked in the exact opposite direction from our home. I knew that Charles needed to continue to work for his own self-worth and sanity. However, every time I mentioned his driving problem to him, he denied it. How could I force him to stop driving?

One day I shared this concern with my boss, Phyllis. I had confided in her about Charles's condition because I felt that she could relate; she was dealing with her son's multiple sclerosis. Phyllis's response was "Why don't you consider getting him a driver?"

As obvious as that sounds now, the idea had not occurred to me. What a huge enlightenment! It gave me hope that Charles could continue working even if he couldn't drive. Now I just needed to wait for the right opportunity to talk to him about it.

It wasn't long before Charles had an accident that got his attention, giving me the opening I'd needed. One day when he was pulling the car into a parking space at work, he didn't see the big green van parked in the spot next to his. He sideswiped the van as he pulled in. The green paint on the side of our champagne-colored Ford Taurus gave it all away.

The fact that he didn't even see the van scared him. When I confronted Charles, he finally confessed that driving *had* become a problem. Then he admitted, "My neuropsychologist told me a few months ago that I should stop driving, but I didn't want to accept it—or tell you." This acknowledgment made me feel upset and relieved at the same time—upset that he hadn't told me before, but relieved that a professional, whom he would be more apt to listen to, had confirmed that he should stop driving. I wondered whether, if the neuropsychologist had told me directly about this recommendation, we could have gotten Charles off the street earlier, reducing the chances of his getting hurt or, worse yet, hurting or killing someone else.

"Charles, I think we should try to find a driver for you. I know that it will feel like you are losing a huge amount of independence, but a driver will allow you to get to work safely. Otherwise, you could have an accident; what if you hurt someone else? With your medical condition, you would be fully liable."

He agreed—surprisingly, without too much hesitation. Even though he had faced the fact that he should no longer drive, he still had to make the painful admission to himself that he would now have to rely on someone else. I just felt tremendous relief that he'd accepted the need for a driver before something worse had happened.

Caregiving Affirmation:
Be creative and plan ahead when seeking ways
to ease difficult life transitions.

Under the pretense that Charles merely had a vision problem, Gerard, the brother of one of the secretaries at Web, volunteered to be Charles's driver. Because he was out on disability for a fall that had injured his back, he had the free time. Little did we know that he would provide even greater services for us down the road—and become a friend to Charles in the process.

THEY CALLED IT "CHARLES'S DISEASE"

"You'll never really know what this disease is until an autopsy is done," Dr. Ravin would say. But how could that help us now? Charles needed to know what disease he had so that he could accept it and move forward. Not knowing was tormenting him, so we continued the search for a diagnosis.

New to working with neurological specialists, we naively expected definitive answers. Charles had been concerned that Dr. Ravin might be too busy for him, as he often found it hard to get a timely appointment with her. When he did meet with her, she listed possible diagnoses but never pinned down the disease. Charles requested a referral for a second opinion; he needed to confirm what she was saying, and also, to try and see if others could help diagnose this disease.

One advantage of living in the Boston area was the plethora of great medical institutions. I think we used each one. We not only got a second opinion from Beth Israel Deaconess Hospital (then known as Deaconess Hospital), but we also went to two other prestigious

Boston hospitals, Boston Medical Center and Massachusetts General Hospital, for third and fourth opinions.

Some of the best neurologists in the country reviewed Charles's case. Each one tried to solve the puzzle. They all had their own opinions. Some thought he had PSP and others thought it was CBGD— all in the Parkinson's-plus category. Others threw out weird names of diseases that I certainly hoped were not real contenders. In the end, most admitted that Charles didn't have enough differentiating symptoms to allow them to diagnose his disease. With each visit, though, Charles went in hopeful that he would learn something new.

To help clarify the picture of this disease, Charles visited various neuro-ophthalmologists and neuropsychologists, too.

As Charles sat in a chair with weird gadgets everywhere, one neuro-ophthalmologist asked him to follow with his eyes the pen that the doctor slowly moved in front of him, from left to right and then from right to left. I watched as Charles's eyes moved in a syncopated rhythm, trying to follow the pen. Then, positioning Charles face-first into a large bowl-shaped contraption, the doctor electronically brought objects into view from various angles until Charles pushed a button to acknowledge that he saw each object from his peripheral vision. These tests all confirmed Charles's problem with the movement of his eyes and his growing loss of peripheral vision.

The neuropsychologists wouldn't let me stay for the nearly full day of tests they performed. But from the reports, I learned that they tested Charles's intellect, his vocabulary, and his arithmetic skills. They checked his memory by asking him to name the president of the United States as well as the state governor, which he could do, but he needed prompting to name the vice president. Being a political junkie, Charles shouldn't have needed any assistance. On a test to recall six digits forward and then four of them backward, they reported that in this skill, he was "mildly constricted for age." As part of the language test, the psychologist instructed him to list as many words within sixty seconds as he could that started with the letter S. They labeled his performance as being "severely constricted for age and education" on this test, as he could think of only eight words. Other tests required him to put objects into patterns and to read aloud. He performed well on a few tests, but very poorly on others. What could be happening to the brain of this man with two master's degrees, this valedictorian of his high school class who'd once been found to have an extremely high IQ of 138?

Even armed with the results of these many tests, the various neurologists continued to throw out the same potential diagnoses—PSP, CBGD, and MSA—not yet able to isolate the correct one. "Or maybe it is something we have not yet discovered," some would admit. The fact that no one knew what ailed him continued to torture Charles, destroying his usual optimism.

Nonetheless, Charles was helped by a bit of genius from the senior neurologist at a Boston hospital. When Charles pressed for a diagnosis, the neurologist said, "Let's call it Charles's disease." For some reason, Charles clung to that. Calling it Charles's disease appeased him for a while, giving him comfort. He now had a name for his condition. "The doctor said to call it Charles's disease," he would later tell others, glorying in his illness's uniqueness.

Caregiving Affirmation:
When you're faced with disappointments, focus on
at least one positive thing.

Making the Most of Our Doctor Visits

Charles and I became experts at going to his medical appointments. We learned how to prepare to make the most of the limited time each doctor had, and I learned the special role I could fill while we were with a doctor.

Preparing for Each Doctor Visit—The Symptom Sheet

As Charles's disease progressed, we slowly grew more attentive to changes in his symptoms. Each neurologist we visited needed to know what symptoms Charles was currently experiencing, and what medications he was taking. And Dr. Ravin, who continued to be his primary neurologist, especially needed to know how the medications she prescribed were working and what new symptoms had popped up since the last visit.

That's why we created the symptom sheet (page 59).

At the top of each symptom sheet, we placed Charles's name, as well as the month and year of the visit. Saving the sheet as a file on our computer made it easy to update it for another doctor visit. We improved the format of the sheets over time until they contained four sections—*New Symptoms/Changes in Symptoms, Ongoing Symptoms, Medications,* and *Questions.*

We started the sheet with the *New Symptoms/Changes in Symptoms* section because we felt that provided the doctor with the most important information first. We broke that section into categories such as *Vision, Fine Motor Movements, Balance, Running, Depression,* and *Insomnia.*

After categorizing each symptom, we then listed in bulleted format the new symptoms or changes in symptoms. For instance, in December 1996 we described Charles's vision this way:

- Seeing with double vision when objects are close
- Losses in peripheral vision
- Right eye hurts occasionally
- When tired, has a hard time keeping right eye open

We listed any symptoms that had not changed since the last visit in the *Ongoing Symptoms* section. We felt that the doctors needed to be reminded of these. We formatted this section the way we did the *New Symptoms/Changes in Symptoms* section, using the same categories and then describing the symptoms related to each category. As an example, the December 1996 sheet included these vision symptoms that hadn't changed since the last visit.

- Reading—can't track across the page
- Difficulty in seeing and recognizing objects
- Deterioration of distance vision
- Failure of depth perception

We broke the third section, *Medications,* into two segments: *Current* and *Past.* Though we didn't always include the latter segment, we found this especially helpful in the first few years of the disease. Charles was trying so many drugs, and several were not working. We didn't want his doctors to forget what he had already tried, and we wanted new doctors to understand his full medication history. With each drug listed, we included the dosage given at each time of day— for example, *doxepin—two 10-milligram tablets at bedtime.*

When we first arrived at doctors' offices, the receptionists always asked what Charles's current medications were. The symptom sheet saved us the time and effort of filling out another form and trying to remember what drugs he was taking and what their dosages were.

The final section, *Questions,* provided an opportunity for us to put in writing our burning questions. It ensured that we remembered to ask them, and that the doctors didn't finish exams without addressing them.

The question Charles would ask most often during the first few years centered on the diagnosis: What disease did he have, and how could it be treated? His next question, which he asked at every visit, dealt with his prognosis: How long did he have to live? (Even though Charles wanted to know the answer to that one, I'm thankful that most doctors didn't answer it in a concrete way.) We often asked questions about medications, such as whether to increase the dose of a medication that was working, or whether to stop taking a drug that was making him spacey. And we always asked about new treatment options or explanations of tests that he had undergone.

The symptom sheets really did help.

In my job at Blue Cross Blue Shield of Massachusetts, I've often heard doctors complain about patients who bring in a long list of questions. My experience with all of Charles's doctors, however, was that they appreciated our symptom sheet. It saved them time because they could more quickly get to solutions instead of just spending much of the visit getting information from us. It allowed the doctors to quickly see Charles's changes. And it provided needed documentation for Charles's medical records. I noticed that for the first few visits, before we started using the symptom sheet, Dr. Ravin seemed to give us just a normal amount of information. But once we used our forms, she started having more in-depth conversations with us.

S Y M P T O M   S H E E T

NAME:_____

DATE: _____

New Symptoms/Changes in Symptoms

New Symptoms
-
-
-
-

Changes in Symptoms
-
-
-
-
-

Ongoing Symptoms
-
-
-
-
-

Medications

Current
-
-
-
-
-

Past
-
-
-
-
-

Questions
-
-
-
-
-

As you can imagine, it was an effort for us to constantly update the symptom sheet. Our lives were busy enough just managing the disease and arranging to keep the doctors' appointments. But the time was well spent because the sheets allowed for more quality time with the doctors. In an era when managed care had whittled doctor visits down to just a few minutes, this was essential. We were able to spend forty-five minutes to an hour with each specialist. The sheets helped us make sure we didn't miss anything important during that precious time.

An unexpected benefit of the symptom sheets was that they allowed Charles and me to have important conversations that would otherwise have been difficult. He didn't always want to tell me what new losses he was facing or what new symptoms had emerged. But filling out the symptom sheets together made it more comfortable for him to be honest with me. The process allowed us each to talk about the symptoms we had noticed, from our own points of view. We could then come to a consensus about what was most important to mention to the doctors.

Caregiving Affirmation:
Use a symptom sheet to communicate more openly
with each other and with your physicians.

At the Visit

Charles and I each had our own role at the doctor's office. Charles was completely the patient. He allowed the doctor to poke and prod, and he answered all the questions asked.

I was the note taker. I'm sure we would have forgotten many of the explanations and instructions if I hadn't jotted them down on the spot. I also asked clarifying questions when I didn't understand something or felt that Charles didn't yet comprehend a doctor's explanation. My background in health promotion proved very helpful, as I had an understanding of the scientific processes. I would have liked to have had a friend or family member who was a nurse accompany us on these visits, but that wasn't possible.

With our mounting experience in the medical system, Charles and I could now effectively work with any physician.

CHARLES FINALLY TELLS OTHERS

"A stranger in the restroom today asked me if I had had a stroke," Charles said to me in a bewildered voice one evening after work. "Can you tell by looking at me that something is wrong?"

Everyone had noticed that Charles had some type of condition, but no one had asked him directly until this stranger did. For months, people had been cornering me when Charles wasn't around to ask me what was happening to him. I tried diplomatically to not say too much. We really didn't know with finality what condition plagued him, and Charles was still adamant that we not tell others.

Until this incident in the restroom, Charles thought he had skillfully hidden his disease from others. As obvious as his condition was, he honestly didn't think others noticed. But now he had to start facing the reality. We talked about how we would officially tell our family, friends, and coworkers.

We started by calling his parents and then both brothers. Charles's younger brother, Ken, expressed sorrow as well as disappointment that he hadn't been told earlier. His chance to be a part of Charles's adult life was suddenly threatened. Ken regretted that they hadn't developed a stronger bond sooner, and immediately committed to getting closer to Charles.

We officially told everyone in my family; although most had already learned about Charles's condition through the family grapevine, now they had the freedom to talk about it with Charles directly.

With great trepidation, Charles told his colleagues at the corporate office at Web Industries. Throughout the course of this disease, he'd been petrified, thinking that once they knew, they would ask him to resign. Instead, they embraced the chance to accommodate his needs in whatever ways they could.

I remember Charles coming home from dinner with Bob Fulton, his company's founder, the night he'd planned to tell Bob about his disease. Charles relayed to me Bob's graciousness and then his admonition: "Charles, I hope this will make you better, not bitter."

This aptly described Charles's hardest fight with this disease—to not let it get him down.

Charles then meticulously worked on a personal letter to inform all two hundred or so employees of the company about his condition. One evening, he brought home the printed letters, labels containing home addresses, and envelopes. Though it was taxing for him, he signed each letter himself, instead of having his signature mechanically reproduced.

"I'm writing to you as a friend—as well as a fellow employee of Web Industries," the letter began. "Over the past year I have been struggling with a health condition that has mystified my doctors." He continued by describing how the disease had affected his vision, causing him to bump into things and making it hard to move his eyes from line to line to read.

After mentioning PSP, which by then we believed to be the proper diagnosis, he explained, "Janet and I are still trying to understand what this diagnosis means. The first word of the name, *progressive*, indicates that it is a condition that gets worse over time. *Supranuclear* refers to the part of the brain that is affected, which is the area that controls the movement of the eyes. And *palsy* is another word for paralysis, meaning that my eyes are locking up."

He went on to admit that it had been hard for him to accept what was happening, and that he even went through a period of depression when he could no longer drive his car. It encouraged me, though, to read one particular sentence he wrote: "My wife has been a wonderful support through this, telling me to focus on my *abilities*, not my *disabilities*."

I wrote in each person's first name on the letter after the *Dear*, and then matched each letter with its label and put it in an envelope.

By waiting so long to tell others, Charles had missed key opportunities for encouragement and support. Now, more than a year after his first symptoms had appeared, he'd finally gone public—and the support poured in.

Charles's brother Ken called every weekend. My family kept in close contact. Friends from his executive MBA program from Georgia State University stepped up their communication with

Charles, writing letters, e-mailing, and calling. The local employee ownership community, in which Charles had a leadership role, continued to make Charles feel special and needed.

Charlie, the fun-loving sales manager at the Atlanta plant that Charles had once managed, took a tape recorder around to the employees there. Many, from Laos, India, and other countries, sweetly shared in their broken English the impact Charles had had on them, and wished him well. What a special tape for him to listen to when he felt down!

E-mails and letters arrived from employees at the other plants, expressing empathy. These people, too, told of how Charles had affected their lives—whether it was their jobs, their family life, going back to school, or accomplishing other self-improvements, Charles had made an impact.

Charles's colleagues at the corporate office graciously accommodated his needs. Sharon, one of the administrative assistants, helped Charles with his reports. Another assistant helped him with everyday needs, such as making sure he got his lunch. The president and other vice presidents provided their reports to Charles in a format he could read. In every way possible, they assured him that he still had a place at Web. Such a compassionate response quickly extinguished his fears of being fired.

Caregiving Affirmation:
Capitalize on opportunities as they arise
and as your loved one is ready for them.

MY COMMITMENT TO STAYING POSITIVE

THE DEMANDS OF CAREGIVING

Even at this early stage, the demands of caregiving started to mount. My time quickly became a slave to this disease, as did Charles's.

All of the household responsibilities fell on my shoulders because Charles could no longer help with the cooking and cleaning. Doctors' appointments required time away from work, which included spending at least an hour in the waiting room before even seeing the doctor. And our free time was eaten up by the most important activity on our to-do list—searching for any information we could find to help us understand this condition.

I struggled with balancing my time better. I determined to cut my hours at work down to forty hours a week. Because this was not my typical work style, I really struggled to not feel guilty about my new 8:30-to-4:30 schedule. But it was the only way to have enough quality time with Charles and the extra time required for caregiving. Nonetheless, dealing with both the known and the unknown issues of this strange disease quickly drained our energy.

Our different ways of handling all of these stressors challenged our relationship in new ways. I was overwhelmed by the increasing responsibilities, even as I struggled to grasp that this was actually happening to Charles. He continued to suffer an intense sense of loss because he could no longer do all the things he'd once taken for granted. At times it felt like an emotional roller coaster—often much more difficult than the physical demands.

But I was committed to making the best of it . . . and our marriage had a strong foundation to help us through.

THE NATURE OF OUR RELATIONSHIP
On a perfect fall day in New England, October 19, 1980, the leaves on the trees were a gorgeous array of orange, red, yellow, and gold. At our small, informal wedding inside the historic 1714 Old Town Meeting House in Lynnfield, Massachusetts, Charles and I recited the vows we had written. Midway through the service, we faced each other at the front of the quaint hall. Charles spoke first:

> *Today, Janet, I give you my life. And before these people, I promise to love you as I love myself. I offer today my unwavering friendship both in the trivial details of life and in the times of crisis.*
>
> *I pledge to support you in your deeper values, to hold you to your better self, and to help you become all that you want to be.*

I offer you the room to flourish as an individual, but with the assurance that you are never alone. Your tears shall be my tears, and your joy my reason for rejoicing. Whatever I am, whatever I have, is yours.

And forsaking all others, I take you to be my wife for as long as we both shall live.

I followed with my vows:

Charles, I love you. Our relationship started out as a deep friendship. I promise to always be your best friend, one you can always trust and count on.

Then, as we started to pursue a romantic relationship, we promised to be good for each other. That promise is still my theme. I will help you to grow as a person. I will support you. I will help you reach the goals that you would like to attain . . .

Our strength as a couple has been our ability to communicate. I promise to always be honest with you and to share my feelings with you so that our relationship will never go stale.

Charles, I promise to never leave you. I will hurt with you, laugh with you, share with you, care for you, and always love you. Forsaking all others, I take you to be my husband.

Throughout our life together, these themes remained strong. We each had our individual lives, but we also remained very close as a couple. We both focused on helping each other be better people and reach our personal and joint goals. Now with this terrible disease, it was imperative that we follow through on that promised support for each other.

Charles reinforced his love for me and our continued commitment to each other on our tenth anniversary, in 1990. What a surprise it was when, after a romantic dinner at a posh Atlanta restaurant to celebrate this milestone, he brought out a ragged folder that was labeled *Janet*. Inside the folder was a bunch of yellow lined paper on which Charles had logged our first dates, fifty-one of them, spanning May 12, 1979, to February 16, 1980. For each one, he'd noted where we went, what we did, and the significant topics we'd talked about.

And it revealed how our growing friendship had developed into a romantic relationship:

- Entry 2, May 19—*dinner at Valles Restaurant*
- Entry 4, June 15—*Ray Charles concert*
- Entry 6, July 2—*walking around the Boston Public Garden*
- Entry 16, September 14—*first kiss*
- Entry 51, February 16—*I am deeply in love with her—intense joy and tinges of sadness. There doesn't seem to be enough time.*

Not only did Charles record these dates, but he also saved the scripts of some of the calls he was about to make to me. Yes, that's right. He actually wrote out ahead of time what he planned to say. I chuckled when I read the notes for his very first call to ask me for a date: "Say, I've decided—especially after talking to you the other evening—that I'd like to get to know you better. I know you're a busy person—every minute is tightly scheduled. But I wonder—could I take you out to dinner sometime? Maybe we could spend some time together and maybe get to know each other better. Next week?"

Can you just imagine how touched and special I felt that Charles had saved this sentimental information—and kept it a secret for ten years so that he could surprise me on our anniversary? What an example of Charles's mastery of making me feel great about myself and our relationship.

That same caring and commitment was still present fifteen years after our wedding. Charles attended a Christian men's retreat in 1995. In an attempt to convert Charles, who had by that point professed to be an agnostic, Dennis, one of the other managers at Web Industries, had begged him to consider going to the retreat. He finally agreed to go. The event's organizers had asked each participant's friends and family to write letters sharing what that person meant in their lives. I wrote to Charles:

> . . . *Our life together has been very special. We really are the lucky ones. But the main reason we have such a wonderful relationship is because of you. You are so selfless—almost too much—that I have all my needs taken care of—by you. . . . I guess the thing I treasure the most is your constant love and commitment to me. It provides deep inner peace to know your love for me—and your loyalty to our relationship. . . . That loyalty allows my self-esteem to flourish—and I become a better person.*

In addition to these special events, Charles and I enjoyed our closeness every day—walking hand in hand, talking through each other's problems, snuggling close together at night, and just plain being affectionate.

KEEPING AN UPBEAT ATTITUDE—REALISTIC OPTIMISM

People asked me if I was angry about Charles's disease. I truly wasn't. Emotionally, I didn't need to know the exact name of the condition and why he had the disease. That's because I consider myself a realistic optimist. My realistic self accepts the fact that life isn't fair. My optimistic self tries to make the best of it all—the proverbial "when life gives you lemons, make lemonade" approach. Keeping a positive attitude didn't mean I always avoided pain—being a caregiver takes an emotional toll. I guess my attitude just gave me the strength I needed to handle the pain.

Charles had so much to give to this world—and he was committed to giving it. It was *not* fair that at the age of forty-five, his body would cave in to a disease that would curtail that giving. Because of my scientific knowledge and my realism, I accept that diseases, accidents, and misfortune happen—randomly—to good people *and* bad. It's just life.

People seem to idealistically believe that medicine and technology should have all the answers. They expect cures, treatments, and solutions when a disease strikes them. And when those easy answers don't come, they blame doctors, whom they think are incompetent. I recognized, however, that the world's scientific and medical knowledge was not advanced enough, especially regarding brain research, to diagnose all diseases correctly and to have the technology and medications to effectively treat all of them. I believed there was more that science and medicine did not know than that it did know. Charles's disease was merely one example, so I accepted that. It would have been normal to feel bad for myself. But somehow I knew that doing so all the time would only lead to a constant spiraling down and down, sucking me into depression like water down a drain. And that kept me from going there.

Then my optimistic side kicked in. I became keenly focused on helping Charles live life as best he could with what he still had left. Maybe a little of my optimism came from having been a cheerleader in high school and college. Back then, I'd enthusiastically cheered on teams even when they'd had no chance of winning.

I've realized over the years that being positive is just part of who I am. But I didn't have this self-awareness earlier on. During college in Nashville, Tennessee, I clearly remember the pretty female classmate with blondish-brown hair who accused me of being a hypocrite. "You can't really be that positive," she blurted out one day as we were each picking up our mail at the student center. Was her out-of-the-blue comment prompted by my typical cheery hello? We were not close friends, but we'd lived in the same dorm and had been pleasant to each other before that incident.

For days after, though, her allegation had haunted me. Was I really just a hypocrite? Was I faking being happy and upbeat? Is it really impossible for someone to keep such a positive attitude? After some agonizing, I finally decided that being cheerful and positive was truly my nature. It is just how I react to the world around me.

In keeping with the cheerleader I had been, I was determined to encourage Charles until he lost his final game. I wasn't consciously aware that our wedding vows were being tested; I was simply committed to helping him have the best possible "rest of his life."

Nonetheless, I felt tremendous sadness on Charles's behalf, watching him trudge through this excruciating emotional struggle and physical decline. I also faced my own deep sorrow at losing Charles bit by bit. But I had no one at whom to be angry. I couldn't blame Charles. It wasn't his fault. And I accepted the fallibility of science and medicine, so I couldn't place the blame on doctors.

In addition, at this point in my life I no longer had the faith in God that I'd once had. Though I still held close the principles from my life of faith—such as forgiving others, giving grace, turning the other cheek, loving your enemies, and not judging others—I didn't believe in God any longer. Around the time Charles and I started to date, I had begun to question how much God intervened in the world. Prior to that, I had believed that God was controlling everything in my life— that He had a plan and was making that plan happen.

But I had begun to doubt this faith when I got a letter from my sister Sue saying, of all things, that God had helped her remember not to burn the Cream of Wheat on the stove. Did God get that involved in our lives? Did He care about the cereal burning? What about all the other times my sister and I had burned food on the stove? Did God not care to intercede then? And if He didn't inter-vene there, did He intervene at all? How could you draw the line to say He didn't do that but He did do this? Finally, I wondered whether He even existed.

At this same time, I was also reading a book on the comparison of the major religions—Christianity, Judaism, Islam, Buddhism, and Hinduism. How could all these cultures and people see God in such different ways—some believing they had the only "true" way? Maybe religion and faith are things humans use to explain the wonders and unknowns of the world they live in. Maybe none of these religions is really true.

By the time disease struck Charles, I had drifted completely away from any faith, so I couldn't blame God or even Satan, whom I also did not believe in, for our tragedy. I couldn't be angry at beings that I no longer believed existed.

And if Charles, the medical system, God, or Satan couldn't be blamed, who could be? Blame was not an option.

Because of the special person Charles was, the charming relation-ship we had, and my innate outlook, I could tackle this disease with a positive attitude. Also, with Charles's remaining time dwindling, I realized that at this moment, his health was as good as it would ever be. His physical condition would only worsen. I was ready to make the best of each day we had together, focusing on spending time doing things that were important and memorable, no matter how exhausted we got.

Caregiving Affirmation:
A positive attitude will provide strength to
help you handle emotional pain.

3

❦

1997: The Losses Accelerate

THE THREAT OF SPEECH LOSS

"Janet, what will I do if I lose my speech?" Charles asked, not really
expecting an answer, one night as we nestled into bed. "I'd have nothing left. I wouldn't be able to continue my mission to help others."

The potential of losing the ability to speak scared him the most.
How would he continue to coach and mentor people at work?
How would he continue to support his friends with caring pep
talks? How would he continue to express his thoughts eloquently,
asking the right questions and giving sound advice? And beyond
his daily communication needs, how would he be able to continue
his public speaking?

Over the years, Charles had displayed a genuine talent for giving a
speech. He could passionately present the issues in which he
believed. This ability was apparent when he was quite young. In high
school, when most of us wanted to hide from teachers who might
ask us to stand up before the class, Charles was winning challenges
on the debate team and spending his Sunday mornings preaching at
small churches in Arkansas.

After college, he preached for a year at a church in Jackson,
Mississippi. He taught thought-provoking college-level philosophy
classes while he worked on his doctoral degree. Then after switching

to a career in business, Charles started doing public speaking at employee-ownership conferences in the United States and abroad.

John, one of Charles's colleagues, likes to share a beautiful example of the impact of Charles's presentations. In 1994, the Shared Participation Foundation of Hungary invited both Charles and John to speak at their employee-ownership conference. It would be attended by managers from companies run by the former Communist regime. John describes the participants as stoic—not responding positively or negatively to any of the speeches, including his own. Though they were polite, their deadpan faces showed neither emotion nor much interest.

But then Charles spoke. "He spent the first ten minutes praising the beautiful city of Budapest that he had been exploring over the last day or so," John said. "He also extolled the virtues of the people of Budapest, and said how much he was enjoying his trip. Then Charles talked with passion about employee ownership at his company, Web Industries. The Hungarian business audience responded to Charles with visible enthusiasm. They even gave him a standing ovation."

Charles always seemed to connect to his audience, and his speaking provided an important avenue for him to share his philosophies. The fear of losing this ability devastated him.

His worst fears were realized when he spoke at *Inc.* magazine's national business conference in 1997. He'd always received glowing evaluations in the past, but this time they were terrible. Visibly depressed, he said, "Janet, I'm a failure. Would you listen to the tape of my talk and tell me what you think? Was I really that bad?"

We put the tape in the car's cassette player and I listened to his painfully slow speech. The concepts that had come across enthusiastically in the past now dragged. I wondered if the disease had caused this, or, instead, the various drugs he was taking. But the cause didn't matter. Charles had just received the lowest blow he could have imagined. In my anxiety about what to say, I simply responded, "It sounds fine to me. You must have just had a difficult audience." But no amount of my trying to sugarcoat the situation could help. Though I felt terrible for him, this new realization was worse for Charles—it was a shock. He couldn't hold back the depression it caused. He kept repeating, "I'm a failure."

As time passed, he began to find it difficult to enunciate his words clearly, and his speech continued to slow even more. By midyear, his speech had started to slur. The progression was inevitable, but the question remained: How would Charles communicate if he couldn't talk?

Caregiving Affirmation:
Despite your support, your loved one may still feel depressed.
Know that this is natural.

A CHALLENGE TO INDEPENDENT RUNNING

After his most recent fall, Charles wouldn't be doing any more running on city streets lined with beautiful houses and elegant landscaping. I wanted to be able to see him at all times while he was running, so we began going to the black cinder track outside Newton's North High School. At the track, I would jog, too, but only every other day. I didn't have the daily commitment that Charles had. On my nonrunning days, I sat on the cement bleachers and plugged away at work projects, peeking up every now and then to keep an eye on Charles.

One day when I wasn't looking, Charles fell. Luckily, he wasn't scraped too badly. I couldn't imagine how he had tripped on the track, with nothing there to trip on. And if he hadn't tripped on something, what had caused his fall? Though this concerned me, our choices for getting in Charles's three miles each day were narrowing, so we continued our daily trek to the track.

Then I saw what had been happening. On a beautiful sunny day, I was jogging at my own pace. When I had finished my laps, I turned to watch Charles. For someone with so many physical losses, he still ran gracefully. But then all of a sudden, he started lifting his knees high, twisting about as if he was stumbling. This awkwardness threw him off balance, and down he went.

A boy about eight years old who also saw Charles fall came running to help. He asked, very puzzled, "Why did he fall?" He recognized, as I had, that Charles could not have tripped on anything.

It looked as if Charles had, for an instant, gotten overwhelmed with fear that he was going to fall, and then did. What is clearer to me now is why some of the neurologists had marveled about Charles's running. They explained that while Charles was losing his ability to make movements at will, he could still do things that were more automatic, which, remarkably, included his running. With that tumble, Charles might have experienced a short circuit of sorts. Maybe he had allowed his thoughts and fears to surface, taking him off automatic pilot and putting him on manual control—exactly what his body could no longer do.

Now, even running on a track was hazardous. He could no longer run on his own. Tremendously disappointed, he agreed that I would need to hold his arm and run with him from that time forward. Although this took away his running independence, it would allow us to once again jog on the beautiful city streets. Much prettier scenes awaited us because we were no longer trapped on the track.

Caregiving Affirmation:
Use your creativity in finding solutions to new challenges.

FACING HAZARDS AT HOME

SHOWERING

Kerplunk—there was that feared sound. I heard it and ran to the shower. Charles was on the floor, twisted in the shower curtain, which fortunately broke his fall, giving him only a few bruises.

Lately I had been assisting him in and out of the shower—helping him step over the old tub's unusually high side. Once in, though, he had been able to take his showers without incident. But not this time. And never again standing on his own.

This time, though, we had been lucky. The 1930s tub in the master bedroom did not have a wall at the foot, so it needed a special shower-curtain rod. The rod, bolted to the wall at the front and rear, also had a smaller metal extension attaching the rod to the ceiling at the curved rear section. Fortunately, this setup provided more support than the typical expandable shower rod would have. The screws pulled partway out when Charles fell, but the rod stayed up. Our top

priority that day was visiting the medical supply store in town to buy
a shower chair. This first of our purchases of aids designed for the
handicapped became another sign of his advancing losses.

FRUSTRATION
"Charles, I'll be right back after I'm dressed to help you to the
kitchen," I said as I helped him sit in the sturdy wooden chair in the
bedroom after getting him dressed. By this time, his disease had progressed to the point where he needed someone to hold his arm even
while he walked.
"I don't need your help," he said. "I can walk over there."
"No, you can't," I said quickly. "You'll fall if you try to walk on
your own."
"No, I won't," he yelled back, hoping that his confidence would
translate into ability.
"Yes, you will. Don't try it, or you *will* fall," I said with ever-
increasing panic in my voice.
"I can walk on my own!" he shouted back defiantly. And then he
tried it. I hadn't been able to talk him out of it. In the belief that
he could just will his body to walk, he got up from his chair. He
took just two or three steps, and then *plop*—down he went. Within
seconds, I was there to pick him up as he sobbed in total frustration at this latest defeat.

EATING
By the time Charles got the fork to his mouth, much of the food
had landed on his lap or the floor, unless it luckily slipped silently
back onto his plate. Because of progressive problems with his depth
perception as well as with coordination, he couldn't easily gather
food on his fork or always successfully get it to reach his mouth. But
he was not willing to accept my help. He refused to be fed like a feeble nursing-home resident. If I tried, he would protest. But I found
it difficult to watch him struggle, dropping food everywhere and taking an unbearable amount of time to finish his meal. Every now and
then, I couldn't restrain myself and would insist on helping him. But
he would object even more strongly: "I can do it myself."

Thankfully, he adapted without complaint, switching to a large soup spoon, which allowed him to scoop his food more easily. And we learned that he did best with food that he could pick up with his fingers—like a piece of bread or his favorite low-fat chocolate sandwich cookies.

When we were alone, it really wasn't a big problem. It just took a long time for Charles to eat, losing some food on the floor in the process. But when we had dinner guests, I felt I needed to do something. We ate at the dining-room table, which sat on top of our expensive handmade burgundy wool rug that had delicate roses at the corners. I wanted Charles to have the dignity he insisted on, but how was I to keep the rug from getting ruined? I quietly placed towels on the floor around his chair without his noticing.

I was also embarrassed by Charles's eating difficulties when we went out to one of our favorite restaurants, such as India Paradise or Appetitos, which we still did quite frequently. Though I found it hard, I had to accept his wishes and just let him struggle and make a mess. But I couldn't understand how Charles felt more dignity eating on his own—spilling food and missing his mouth—than when I helped neatly feed him. Finally, I realized that maintaining some independence motivated Charles even when it didn't seem logical.

Unreliable Brain Signals

"I instinctively now reach for things with my left hand," Charles said, describing how the disease had aggressively attacked his right side. "And I always lead with my left foot when I start walking." Because he was right-handed, losing the ability to use his right side effectively further complicated his life . . . and mine. He required total assistance for getting dressed and even for rolling over in bed periodically throughout the night.

We also noticed what is called an action tremor, or intention tremor. At that point, Charles didn't have a persistent tremor like you might see in someone with Parkinson's disease, such as actor Michael J. Fox. But when Charles started to move—such as to stand up or reach for something—his body or hand shook.

Occasionally, Charles even had tremors when he sat still. The first time this happened, it nearly scared me to death! And it frightened Charles, too.

Sitting on the shower chair one morning, Charles yelled, "Ahhhhhhh!"

"What is it?" I called from the adjacent bedroom, hurrying in to see what was happening. Charles's leg was bouncing uncontrollably up and down, causing his foot to slap the shower floor on each bounce. He couldn't make it stop. I helped him finish his shower and wrapped him in a fluffy towel, hugging him tight to help calm the tremor. Thankfully, the leg-bouncing and foot-slapping happened only a few more times, but not before showing us what—not who—was in charge of Charles's body now.

His brain pulled other cruel tricks. One oddity was that Charles's arm would just float up in front of him. He wouldn't notice that it was out of place. When this happened, I'd gently put it down by his side.

And then one day, Charles admitted to me on one of our jogs: "I can't do math anymore."

"What do you mean, you can't do math? What is three plus five?" I asked, assuming this would be easy.

To my astonishment, he replied, "I don't know."

"Two plus two?" No response.

Later, when we talked to Dr. Ravin, she acknowledged that math skills tend to be the first to go when the brain's mental functions are affected. Neither of us expected this loss, which then had me questioning what cognitive skill would go next. At every corner, Charles faced disappointments and losses that tore at his positive attitude. He became a frustrated optimist, trying hard to keep upbeat but always teetering on the edge of depression.

Caregiving Affirmation:
Allow your loved one to maintain independence
in daily tasks as much as possible.

TRIP TO ISRAEL: RECOGNIZING THE LOSSES

"You have to go," Charles told my mother when she called one day from her home in Florida. She had just mentioned to him that she was thinking about going to Israel with a group from her church. "Some of my friends have taken this trip in the past and have raved about it," she said. After my father's death, Charles had actively encouraged my mother to travel and to not hold back from doing things she enjoyed. "What a fabulous opportunity. You won't want to miss out on this adventure," he added passionately. Then, without her asking, he invited us on the trip, too.

So on a beautiful day in May 1997, Charles and I flew from Boston to John F. Kennedy International Airport in New York. Claiming our bags at one terminal in JFK, we lugged them onto a shuttle bus to the El Al terminal. With Charles's instability in walking, and my having to handle all of our luggage within the tight transfer time allowed, we both were exhausted and frantic when we finally arrived at the departure gate only minutes before takeoff. Then to my astonishment, with Charles barely able to stand on his own next to me, the attendants commanded me to open every piece of luggage and show the contents all the way to the bottom. I felt like they were picking on me, and I couldn't understand why, because they could clearly see Charles's dilemma. I later learned that this in-depth scrutiny was normal, and the only way El Al had been able to fly incident-free for so many years. But at the time, it nearly put me into tears. With this much struggle so early on, how could we ever get through this trip?

But finally, we met up with Mom and the full group from Florida at Gatwick Airport in London, where we boarded our plane to continue on to Israel.

Our bus trip started immediately on our arrival in Tel Aviv. Our packed itinerary took us from top to bottom of the entire country, with stops in more than fifteen cities and towns, and many sights to see in all of them.

With both an Israeli and an American guide sharing information with us, we found the trip rich with the history of the ancient land

Charles and I had read about in the Bible earlier in our lives. We
were filled with awe at the depth of the conflict between the cultures
currently living so close together. This struggle became ominously
apparent during our visit when a group of Israeli schoolchildren were
shot and killed on a field trip near the Jordan border. And every time
we saw Israeli schoolchildren at historic sites, bodyguards stood close
by, openly carrying guns.

Trips have a way of making a person much more acutely aware
of lost or changed abilities. Because we took so many trips, they
started to become the markers by which we chronicled the status of
Charles's disease.

On this trip, even with his new glasses, Charles had to struggle
with his eye movements to be able to find and see all the sights.
"Don't ask me that anymore!" he finally said with frustration when I
naively asked, "Charles, did you see that?" one too many times as the
bus whizzed by famous sights.

For Charles, this trip also highlighted the creeping impact of this
disease on his stability and movements. His greatest challenge was in
getting on and off the narrow, steep steps of the bus. A teenage girl
on the trip with us hopped up quickly at every stop to graciously
assist Charles. At first, needing assistance frustrated him. "I can do it
on my own," he'd say, as he almost toppled over in getting his foot to
the first step. The girl and I learned to make this a game with him,
making light of the fact that he was dependent on us, which helped
him quickly adapt to the extra support.

Charles's physical instability also manifested itself as we maneuvered the ancient rocky paths of cities like Megiddo, Jericho, and
Jerusalem. Mom and I each took one of his arms to keep Charles
from falling and lagging too far behind the group.

Our tourist boat trip on the Sea of Galilee started out very calm.
We moved gently across the sea and stopped offshore just before
reaching the ancient ruins of Capernaum. An Israeli dressed in first-
century fisherman's garb had just finished demonstrating the casting
of nets when the sea suddenly turned rough. The "fishermen" tried
docking the boat in Capernaum, but couldn't. So, the boat bobbing
furiously, we headed back across the sea for an inlet where the waters

would be calmer. We moved Charles from the white plastic chairs that had started sliding around the deck to the built-in bench along the sides of the deck. For the entire ride back, my mother and I held him tightly to keep him—and ourselves—from falling to the deck, while others in our party got seasick.

One precious memory I have is jogging with Charles, holding tightly to his arm, through a historic park on the Mount of Olives. The air smelled clean as we ventured around ancient rocks and through desertlike gardens. I don't know if it was the beauty of the park or the awe I felt at the history under my feet that made this experience so special. I felt pleasure and thankfulness that Charles and I could experience the thrill of running together through such a gorgeous and inspiring setting. And I sensed that Charles felt the same.

Charles's favorite place seemed to be the mountaintop fort and palace of King Herod at Masada. Rich with history and mysterious ruins, Masada is where the Jews held out for a number of years before committing mass suicide to escape the invasion of the Romans in CE 73.

As we started the tram ride up, Charles seemed amazed that this civilization had existed at the top of a mountain. As he walked arm in arm with Mom and me, Charles expressed wonder at seeing the remains of the Jews' living quarters: still-beautiful tiles and paintings, storerooms that once held enough food to last for seven years, a technically advanced bathhouse, and cisterns that effectively collected water at the mountaintop from the vast desert that surrounded it. As the group hurried to board the tram at the end of our mountaintop visit, I decided that I just had to run back up to the kiosk and buy Charles a Masada baseball cap, even though it might hold up our group. His eyes gleamed in appreciation when I revealed my purchase to him after we were back on the bus.

Though he enjoyed the trip overall and felt pleased to have had this terrific opportunity, the physical and visual difficulties he experienced made it clear to him that his disease was progressing swiftly. He slept restlessly and sometimes seemed agitated during the day, especially when it was hard for him to keep up with the group and take in sights that for him slipped by too quickly. Some days he just clammed up, saying little and withdrawing into himself. It saddened me that he felt this emotional pain and couldn't get as much pleasure from the trip as he would have if he had been well. And it made me feel somewhat guilty that I so utterly enjoyed myself.

Dealing with the depression that surfaced proved harder for him than the physical challenges of the trip. But the depression only intensified his desire to experience all that he could possibly squeeze into the life left to him.

Caregiving Affirmation:
Take pleasure in every moment you spend together.

OUR EXHAUSTING DAILY ROUTINE

The alarm rang at 5:15 AM, jolting me out of bed. Charles and I put on our tattered sweatpants and worn-out T-shirts, with me assisting him, and then we headed out to jog. Our run took us along Commonwealth Avenue, a tree-lined boulevard with beautiful Victorian homes.

We used our jogging time to practice speech exercises. I'd torn out a couple of pages from Charles's issue of *Time* magazine to use as my prompt. "Project," I said to Charles, reading the word from the magazine article that I held, folded in fourths, in my free hand while supporting him with my other hand. "This *project* is boring," Charles said, putting the word into his own sentence. We'd learned this exercise from my sister Carolyn, a speech therapist, to help Charles practice not only articulation but also the cognitive process of putting words together. When we did the exercise, I needed the magazine prompt because I would get in a rut trying to dream up new words on my own. *Time* provided words like *arbitrary, campaign, influential,* and *embarrassed*—enough to allow me to quiz Charles for nearly the entire jogging route.

The run was the easy part. By the time we'd get home, Charles's body would have stiffened. His head, cocked back, tilted his balance so far backward that I strained to keep him from falling. Standing behind him, my arms under his, I used my entire body weight to block Charles so he wouldn't fall backward as we painstakingly climbed each of the thirty stairs, one by one, to the front door. I often felt panicked during these climbs, and wondered if our jogs were getting too risky.

I knew what came next in our routine. Once we were safely in our bedroom suite after a jog, showering would be the next obstacle to overcome. While I held his arm as firmly as I could, Charles would step over the high rim of the old bathtub. Then we'd maneuver him into a sitting position on the gray-and-chrome shower chair. By this point, he needed assistance washing. We began to use the long hose with the shower nozzle on the end, already installed by the previous owners of the house. I soaped him up, washed his hair, rinsed him off, and dried him.

Once, I'd only done his buttons and tied his tie. Now, my job had expanded to fully dressing him. He couldn't balance himself and use his right hand to coordinate this most basic of daily tasks. He sat and stood, sat and stood as I put on his underwear, shirt, pants, socks, and shoes every morning, then stripped him every night.

It was hard enough for Charles to accept that he needed this degree of assistance. But he found it nearly impossible to admit his growing problem with incontinence. The accidents started with a sudden urge to go and his not always making it to the bathroom in time. And then he began to leak a little after we had already zipped up his pants.

At the time, drugstores sold men's underwear shields to protect clothing from incontinence. When I tried to put these inside his underwear, he'd yell, "I don't need these! Why are you insisting I wear them?"

For many months, every morning I had to coax Charles into wearing them. "You can't tell it's there," I'd assure him. And to make it seem not too out of the ordinary, I'd say, "I wear a panty shield every day, too," which I actually did. "It just gives me confidence—just in case I can't get to the restroom on time," I'd add. My most persuasive argument, I think, was when I told him that this was "just biology" and nothing to be embarrassed about. Nonetheless, it was a fight almost every day.

Charles diligently swallowed all of his new pills. He no longer
took the superantioxidants, continuing to complain that they made
him feel "spacey." He now took the typical antiparkinsonian medication Sinemet. We couldn't tell if it really helped, but at least it didn't
cause any noticeable side effects. He started taking Zoloft for depression, which also didn't appear effective against this strange disease.
But two other drugs did seem to help. One, Ativan, quelled what
had become a frequent complaint: "My feet are hot!" Another one,
called Mirapex, was a *dopamine agonist*, driving dopamine into the
cells, as Dr. Ravin explained. It lessened the number of choking
episodes he had been experiencing when swallowing liquids, and the
slight slurring that had appeared in his speech.

I began to notice that all morning Charles would obsessively and
anxiously ask, every few minutes, "What time is it?" He was constantly worried that we were running late. Was this fixation a new
symptom of his creeping neurological degeneration?

Gerard, Charles's new driver, picked him up every morning, assisted him down the stairs, and then drove him to work in our second
car, the Dodge Aries. Once Charles was out of the house, I had to
get myself showered, dressed, and off to work.

The disease's effects on his vision, movements, and continence
affected his ability to do his job. As the year progressed, he completely lost his handwriting, coming to depend totally on his one-finger
approach to typing on his computer. He also stopped practicing the
eye exercises that Dr. Hammer had given him, realizing that they
didn't improve the accelerated losses. "My right eye tends to drift
outward, and I sometimes see double," he said of another complicat-
ing factor. "I'm not able to track my eyes across a line. And it's hard
to find the next line, too." So as reading the words on the screen
became difficult, he used a larger font size and double-spaced all of
his documents.

Unfortunately, though, the reports generated by people in the
other areas of the company did not use these same techniques. The
financial reports gave him the most difficulty.

"Charles, how are you able to read those reports?" I asked.

He sheepishly replied, "I sometimes have to fake my understand-

ing of them so the other guys won't find out that I can't read them."
He also admitted that he couldn't focus when he looked hard at
something—like telephone numbers. I can't imagine how that felt for
this normally unstoppable high achiever.

Charles also had to deal with his pride about a more basic issue at
the office. Al, the human resources manager, assisted him wherever
he needed to go. Al held Charles's arm, like a sighted person assisting
a blind person, to keep him from bumping into things or falling as
he traveled to the conference room or lunchroom. Al even helped
with all of Charles's trips to the restroom, assisting Charles in unzipping and zipping his pants or pulling them down so he could sit on
the toilet. "I've worked as a medic in the armed services," Al said
once when I thanked him for this most personal help. "I don't find
this uncomfortable," he assured me. But I'm certain that Charles did,
at least at first. Though Charles was a proud, stubbornly independent man, his tenacity couldn't overcome his disability this time. Al's
support, however, provided the only way for Charles to keep working that year, and work was what provided Charles with much of the
meaning he found in life.

In the evenings after work, Charles could no longer cook for me.
We resorted to frozen prepared meals and chili from a can—using
the best of my pitiful cooking skills. At bedtime, Charles would
down the new sleeping pill the doctor had prescribed, which didn't
work any better than the previous one—ending his day with a restless night's sleep.

Caregiving Affirmation:
Expect caregiving demands to increase over time.

DIALOGUE DIFFICULTIES

Apathetic is not a word anyone would have used to describe
Charles. Always engaged in life, Charles tackled everything he faced
enthusiastically. His past experience and skill as a preacher and public debater were why Charles relished intense conversations on topics
he believed in strongly. It probably started with his relationship with

his father. Charles and his dad always debated their religious ideas, masterfully throwing out Bible verses to prove their points.

We had socialized in recent years with people who believed in the liberal ideals of taking care of the disadvantaged. Charles often sparked conversations at our dinner parties revolving around themes of progressive business practices, such as employee ownership, involving workers in company decisions, and implementing team participation. The half dozen or so people sitting around our dining-room table would express their opinions in answer to Charles's leading questions. "How can we get others to understand these values?" he'd ask, prompting more discussion.

Gradually, these energetic discussions became dominated by others. By this point in his disease's progression, Charles mostly listened. His speech had definitely slowed. But it also seemed liked the disease hampered his ability to collect his thoughts. And with the group's conversation whirling in lots of directions, he didn't even try to express his opinions.

We needed to give him time to speak. Initially, I'd stop the dialogue every so often and say, "Charles, what do you think about that?" But even with this invitation, he seemed shy about adding his own input. I felt certain that he wanted to contribute to the discussion, but he just couldn't.

Caregiving Affirmation:
Find ways to include your loved one in events large and small.

Eventually, the cause of his lack of engagement turned from inability to indifference. His mind seemed somewhere else, his face somewhat expressionless. I wondered if he even cared to be a part of the discussions anymore. Had this disease already taken away that wonderfully passionate place in his brain that was so full of ideas and opinions?

LESSONS ON COPING

Ten other people, each with a condition such as chronic fatigue syndrome, severe headaches, and chronic pain, sat in metal folding chairs in a circle with Charles and me. Over the nine-week program, Peg, the instructor, led the group through myriad relaxation exercises and cognitive-behavioral techniques. Charles and the other ten hoped to learn how to cope with their debilitating symptoms, such as sleepless nights and pain.

We were in the stress-reduction program offered by The Mind/Body Medical Institute. Insurance paid for Charles to partici-pate. But I felt lucky when the director invited me to attend with Charles at no cost. It was obvious that I would need to assist him with projects during the class and help him take notes. But with the instructor's encouragement, I, too, got to participate in the exercises.

Peg talked about relaxation as a nonjudging awareness—turning off the inner dialogue to decrease the stress response.

"Breathe in deeply; now exhale slowly," Peg would say softly and deliberately, instructing us in the fifteen-minute relaxation tech-niques. But doing them at home, even with the cassette tapes, seemed to be a chore, and we had difficulty finding the time. One day, though, sitting on the love seat in our breakfast room after din-ner, Charles asked me to perform the exercises on the relaxation tape with him. Peg, in her persuasive way, must have convinced him of the need to try to fit these into our busy schedule. And I think he felt they would help me cope with our stress, too. Taking slow breaths in and out, we practiced the technique we'd been taught.

Unfortunately, though, we didn't continue with the full fifteen-minute exercise much after the class ended. But we did stick with the shorter relaxation exercises that both of us found easier to fit into our busy days. For example, one of them involved simply counting down from ten to zero, taking a deep breath in and out with each number.

During class each week, we recorded whether Charles's symp-toms—depression, loss of visual depth perception, and fatigue—changed for the better or worse. Unfortunately, we saw no improve-ment over the nine weeks. In fact, his symptoms continued to wors-en with the progression of the disease. But the class gave us tremen-dous insight into coping. Peg taught us that with any crisis comes not only danger, but also an opportunity to grow in personal ways. We were experiencing the danger, and Peg was coaching us to find the opportunity.

The techniques that seemed to help Charles and me the most taught us how to change negative thinking, because at this point in the disease's progression, the mounting losses Charles faced were eroding his positive attitude. He kept feeling more and more like a handicapped person, which depressed him. Peg tried to help Charles discover the difference between rational and irrational negative thoughts. If the thoughts were negative but also rational—such as *This disease is getting worse*—she encouraged us to accept this fact and then make meaning out of it. "Concentrate on pleasant thoughts and affirmations. Believe that your lives have meaning and purpose," she said. But if the thoughts were irrational, she'd say, "Change your thinking about them."

To give insight into the irrational negative thoughts, Peg encouraged us to keep track of them in a log. With my help, Charles filled out the log each week. "What stressful event did you experience today?" I'd ask. Charles responded one week with "I felt like I wasted my day." Other times, he said, "I feel like I don't have influence at work" or "I felt handicapped today and got depressed" or "I'm not able to run without help anymore."

"What feelings did you have when facing that stressful event?" I asked next. The words *depressed, frustrated, sense of loss, embarrassed, inadequate,* and *disappointed* would typically be in his response. "What thoughts were you having when you were experiencing those feelings?" the form prompted me to say. And his answers?

"I can't do things I used to do. . . . I can't even type anymore. . . . Even seeing keys on the phone is difficult. . . . I looked at my files and saw all the stuff I used to do and can't do anymore. . . . I might as well give up. I will end up in a wheelchair. . . . I'm going to end up in a nursing home. . . . I have to face the fact that I'm going to die soon."

The hardest part of the exercise came at the end. We had to distinguish between which thoughts were true and which ones were distortions of the truth. Then we had to determine how to change the distortions into more positive responses. For instance, "I can't do a lot these days," which Charles often said, is a "*should* statement," which means it implies that you should be doing something. Making that kind of statement is like scolding yourself, and it's also perfectionism—both doomed to depress you. A more rational and affirming way to restate that "should statement" might be "How can I find meaning in what I can still do?"

Caregiving Affirmation:
Work together to make meaning out of the tragedy of disease.

I used this exercise many times at home, especially on our morning jogs, when Charles would express a negative, destructive thought. Most of the time, Charles seemed to appreciate this reminder. But changing to a more positive way of thinking continued to challenge him. He kept trying to do things he could no longer do, denying that they were now beyond his capability. This just made him angry, irritated, and disappointed. It wasn't that he didn't *want* to change his thinking, but that the disease tugged hard at his optimism, managing to frustrate him at every turn. This was so unlike the upbeat attitude he'd always had.

At our discharge session alone with Peg, she encouraged Charles by saying, "Milk your illness for meaning and purpose, explore being the object of your own mission statement and give yourself grace, and increase your daily pleasures." How wise and right on!

TIME TO MAKE MAJOR LIFE CHANGES?

"Janet, have you thought about quitting your job?" "Should you and Charles think about retiring?" "Is this the time to sell your house and move closer to your family?" "With his clock winding down, what does Charles want to do with the rest of his life?" "Is it time to just live life without the constraints of a job?"

These questions swirled around us from friends and family. We had hit a new juncture in our life. Should we totally uproot? Maintain the status quo? Or slightly modify our goals and ambitions?

Charles clearly wanted to continue to build on the foundations he had already laid in his life—supporting the employees at Web Industries, providing a leadership role in the ESOP Association, and speaking about his caring leadership style at conferences. He wasn't willing to compromise these aspirations. And though being with family would be great, he'd have to leave his very good friends and close connections to do that. Escaping and uprooting were not options for him.

And I agreed. We ignored these questions as long as we could and focused on living our lives as normally as possible.

Caregiving Affirmation:
Periodically reevaluate whether it's time to make major life changes.

FINALLY TIME TO MOVE

THE STAIRS!

Charles loved our dramatic Victorian house set on a hill in Newton. From the first day he walked through the house, he developed a vision for making it our home. Its turn-of-the-nineteenth-century charm only magnified its potential. The charisma drew you in as you entered the front foyer through the gigantic old door with its huge oval glass window and glass doorknobs. Once you were inside, you found a magnificent staircase overlooking the expansive foyer, complete with fireplace and hardwood floors. We could just picture hosting a wedding in the house and having the bride walk down the steps to meet her groom on the rail-enclosed platform at the bottom.

Over the years we had lived there, Charles had made it his dream house. He'd redesigned the kitchen, tearing it down to just the studs. The new kitchen gave us a wonderful cooking area amid classic cherry cabinets with speckled rose and gray granite countertops. The counter peninsula with two stools allowed us an easy place to set up quick dinners. This opened into a sitting area where Charles and I preferred to eat a more leisurely dinner on the comfortable love seat while watching the evening news.

We'd hired a talented decorator, Kay, who finished the rest of our downstairs, adding faux finishes on the walls and beautifully coordinated accessories. We especially loved the bathroom on the first floor tucked three steps down into the circular space of the turret, with stained-glass windows all around. Kay hung wallpaper depicting a Victorian picnic with women in long, flowing dresses playing lawn tennis or holding parasols, and men wearing top hats and holding canes. Her touch helped fulfill Charles's dream for the house.

But now we would have to move. The thirty-plus stairs we had to climb to reach the front door had become impossible for Charles. And then there was getting to the second-floor master bedroom. Taking him up the stairs caused my heart to work harder more from the panic than from the exercise. A few times, Charles's rigidity after our jogs hampered my stability so much that it forced me to take him back down the one or two steps on which we had just struggled. Exasperated, I would put him in the car in the garage and recruit help from Dorin, our Romanian houseguest who had been living with his wife in our third-floor au pair suite for the last year or so.

I felt like Charles's life was in the balance every time we tackled the stairs. What if I lost hold of him or lost my own balance and he and I tumbled down the steps? This frightened me more than almost anything else. The difficulty in getting Charles's stiffened body up the stairs finally became more than I could handle. Charles reluctantly and sadly agreed.

NOW WHERE DO WE GO?

Once we made the decision to move, we both agreed that we desperately wanted to stay in Newton. The access road parallel to Commonwealth Avenue provided a safe running route—one of our top priorities. But most of the houses were two or three stories—like ours, with all the bedrooms and full baths on the second floor. The few ranch-style homes available needed major renovations. The swift progression of Charles's condition wouldn't allow us the luxury of a move and then the disruption of carpenters, plumbers, and electricians.

To our good fortune, a corner lot just down the street from our house and on Commonwealth Avenue came on the market. The owner of a large Victorian house had subdivided his land to produce this lot. Perfect!

After we and the owner signed the purchase and sale (P&S) agreement, we began the arduous work of finding a builder, viewing various plans, and selecting an option. We loved the designs from one builder—but the costs kept creeping higher and higher, making us uncomfortable with this decision in light of the unknown costs that Charles's condition could bring. Then, luckily, the man selling the land started to add new requirements to the P&S, such as insisting we plant particular types of hedges between our property and his. Working with our savvy lawyer, feeling both sadness and relief, we withdrew our bid with no financial penalty.

This caused us to rethink our plans. The suburbs west of Newton offered more affordable housing prices—with a greater inventory of new homes. "Maybe it would be better living farther west and closer to your job," I suggested to Charles. I felt that this would allow his coworkers to visit more easily when he eventually became home-bound. He probably thought only about the shorter commute, not about later visits. He agreed, and we began to look at the western suburbs of Natick and Framingham.

On our first day of searching in Framingham, we found a new home, not quite finished, with a master suite on the first floor. Our hopes rose as we enjoyed the thought of not having to renovate an old ranch. And the price was more favorable than that of any house we could have found or built in Newton. The Framingham house, located less than a mile from the Massachusetts Turnpike, would help out with my commute. And busy Route 9, a half mile from the house, offered us the convenience of its many restaurants, stores, movie theaters, and a shopping mall. We immediately put in an offer that the builder accepted.

Over the next few weeks, we excitedly picked out the light fixtures and carpet colors and then waited anxiously for the closing date in August. But we began to worry when we didn't see the builder making any progress in completing the house. The lighting store didn't even deliver the fixtures. Finally, we learned that the builder was defaulting on his bank loan—not only on this house, but also on about ten other properties in the neighborhood. Neither the bank nor the real estate agent could give us any details. We felt thankful for our lawyer again, who counseled us to not pay the five-thousand-dollar deposit directly to the builder, as originally stated in the P&S, and instead put it into an escrow account. Without that counsel, we would have lost the entire deposit. *Whew!*

We were again forced to start a new search for a house. Unfortunately, nothing we toured compared to the Framingham house. As the summer ended and the fall approached, I determined that we had to find a temporary solution. With Charles's condition progressing quickly, I seriously doubted that we could wait for the default on the Framingham house to be finalized, allowing us to buy it either from another builder or from the bank's auction.

My sister Barb and her husband, Jack, visited at just the right time. They realized our dilemma and searched for an apartment for us. After visiting three or four properties in Framingham, they came home excited to have found just the right one. "It meets your two most important needs—an elevator to get you to the apartment and a walk-in shower," Barb said. She mentioned that it also was furnished and we could rent it monthly. For those privileges, though, the cost would be twenty-five hundred dollars a month. Though it was an astronomical price for a two-bedroom apartment, we had no other choice. Staying in Charles's dream house in Newton was no longer possible.

Barb and Jack helped us complete the deal, and we prepared to move in mid-November. Then we finally heard from the bank. They were putting the Framingham house up for auction. We now had a chance to buy it.

We had one advantage in being able to offer the best bid for this house. We knew its market value, and we knew exactly what work still needed to be done. We talked to our lawyer to determine the maximum price we would offer during the auction.

On a cool fall day in November, Charles and I arrived early and watched two other properties auctioned—one had only a foundation on it and the other was just a lot. Charles found it difficult to stand in one place during each of these auctions. So, holding his arm for support, I walked him around in our own little circles, giving away to those watching that Charles had some sort of physical problem.

By the time of our house's auction, Charles could no longer stand.

I remembered that we had packed his shower chair in the car for our trip to the ESOP Association's meeting of the board of directors in Las Vegas, where I was taking Charles that afternoon. I got it out and sat Charles down on it in the driveway close to the house. I stood behind him, and everyone else participating in the auction gathered around us, facing the bank's auctioneer, who stood just in front of the porch.

The auctioneer originally started the bidding very high. When the group balked, he then brought it lower. I waited as patiently as I could (which was not quite patient enough, I suppose) and countered the offers made. During the auction, I noticed that the man whom someone had pointed out as being the original seller of the land was increasing the amount after each counteroffer I made. And other people who did not look like couples wanting to buy the house were also raising the bids. "Contractors who have lost money with this builder will be trying to push the purchase price as high as possible," our lawyer had warned us before the auction. "They are on a priority list with the bank. Those at the bottom of the list may not get their money back if the house does not sell at a high enough price."

When the auctioneer reached the highest amount we were willing to pay, our lawyer commented loud enough for others to hear, "Isn't that your highest bid?" That was all it took for the others to stop. "Sold!" the auctioneer said to us.

Then the entire crowd burst out with applause. It was comforting to know that they did have some mercy. One of the people who occasionally raised the bid congratulated us and said that he was losing tens of thousands to this builder and was not going to recoup it on this house. But he did not want to raise the bid any higher, for our sakes. Revealing, in the softness of his voice, how much this touched him, our lawyer commented that he had never seen people clap after an auction. He then worked quickly to coordinate the closing—scheduling it for mid-December along with the one for our Newton house.

Once we bought the Framingham house, I reluctantly moved into the role of general contractor, as some major work still needed to be completed. I would have to coordinate the final projects, as well as obtain the occupancy permit from the town. The town conservation committee required us to finish the basic landscaping and seeding, but finally conceded by allowing a temporary permit until spring.

And that was only the start of the overwhelming management required. I located a carpenter to install a ramp in the garage. It would make it easier for Charles to get in and out of the house—and to eventually accommodate a wheelchair. The carpenter also mounted handrails in the bathroom, next to the toilet, and in and around the shower. We brought Kay, our decorator, back to have the plain off-white walls throughout the downstairs painted in our favorite pastel colors—as well as add some special touches with stencils and hand-painting. That alone made the house feel like our own. We also decided to change the Formica countertops in the master bath to Corian, and the ones in the kitchen to granite.

We expected all this work to take at least another month. Therefore, we had to move into the apartment that Barb and Jack had found for the short term, meaning that we had to pay rent on the apartment as well as the mortgage for the new house. All of this responsibility brought me to tears of frustration a number of times. I felt angry that no one could help me. It was all on my shoulders. How could I manage all of these tasks, continue to go to work each day, care for Charles's increasing needs—which included coordinating his rides to work, dressing him, and taking him for his runs—and still keep spirits high in both of us? Able or not, I just did it.

Caregiving Affirmation:
No matter how overwhelmed you both are, make a
commitment to keep your spirits high.

PREPARING TO MOVE

If you have ever moved, you know the torture—finding a mover, packing, canceling utilities, changing phone numbers, and on and on. Most of us would rate the cumulative annoyance level of these tasks as worse than that of a root canal. Add to that caring for a husband handicapped by a neurological disease, and you can begin to imagine the tremendous stress that I faced.

Friends and family, however, came to our aid.

My staff at Blue Cross Blue Shield and Charles's friend June kept insisting on helping in some way. So we planned a "packing and cleanup" party with them one Saturday. I furnished the pizza and drinks; they supplied the manual labor. Dressed in their chore-time jeans and T-shirts, a few packed all the books throughout the house—not a small task, because Charles was such an avid reader. The others lugged pieces of lumber and junk left by the previous owner from under the front porch and in the basement to a Dumpster outside. They all went home exhausted, not surprising when I figured out that they contributed a whopping forty person-hours of work to our efforts.

My family also wanted to help. Kay, our decorator, had painted the downstairs and our master bedroom and bath, but we still had two bedrooms, an extra bath, and upstairs hallway to finish. We could not sell the house as it was—especially because a couple of years earlier, my sister Carolyn and her husband Tony had helped us start stripping the old dark green Victorian-looking wallpaper from the second- and third-floor hallway, and we'd never finished it. Also, one night Charles had wanted to see what was behind a piece of gypsum board that replaced the old horsehair plaster in a section of hallway just outside our bedroom door, so he'd smashed a hole in the board . . . only to find nothing of importance. At a minimum, we needed to fix that and the half-removed wallpaper before putting the house on the market.

All of my sisters, two brothers-in-law, and my brother flew in from various parts of the United States to donate a week to do the work.

Sue arrived first and found some heavy-duty wallpaper to put on the main wall of the second-floor hallway. It would hide all the bumps and blemishes, covering the old wallpaper, the gypsum board, and the hole she patched. She worked two days to get that project completed. Then, like a drill sergeant, she coordinated the rest of the crew. Each member had an assigned task.

My sisters did the meticulous painting of the stairway spindles as well as the woodwork and walls in the bedrooms. In addition to wallpapering and painting the extra bathroom upstairs, the guys handled the steamer and scraped off the old, limp wallpaper throughout the massive second- and third-floor hallways. Above one doorway the freshly removed wallpaper revealed a date written on the plaster—JUNE 5, 1905—confirming the house's hundred-year-old history. Charles and I felt deeply disappointed when the next day we saw that someone had rolled wall paint over the historic date. We were upset that we hadn't clearly shared our interest in somehow preserving it.

Charles and I left each morning to go to our jobs. When arriving home, we loved seeing our family members' progress and especially enjoyed our evening meals with them. We had fun-loving conversations, laughing and enjoying each other. Charles mostly listened but would laugh heartily with the rest of us. The week went by without even having the occasional family spat.

Within a week, they completed all the work—contributing another three hundred person-hours to the project. We cataloged the effort with pictures, including a final shot of the workers posed in front of their finished handiwork. I didn't realize until I developed the pictures how big a risk Tony and Doug, my brother, had been taking in standing on a makeshift scaffold—teetering three levels up over the three-story stairway—to reach the ceiling of the third-floor hallway with paintbrushes attached to broom poles. The scaffold also held them as they completed the steaming and scraping of the old wallpaper and rolling new paint on the high stairway walls.

With the renovations complete, we could now hire a realtor. As with the first house we owned in Atlanta, we interviewed three realtors to determine which one we liked best. Before long, we had selected one, and she quickly put the house on the market. We expected the house to sell quickly, as it was a seller's market. But we learned over time that though people loved the house, the stairs were as much a deterrent for them as they had become for us.

Our fears mounted when the house didn't sell during the vigorous spring selling season. After lowering the price, we finally got a serious offer in the fall. The buying couple currently lived in the Back Bay of Boston but wanted to move to the suburbs to start a family. Living on the third floor of a triple-decker, they were used to trekking stairs each day. Interestingly, I found out that our buyers were best friends with one of the writers I worked with at Blue Cross.

Finding movers and packers was our next task. My mother timed her next visit to help us interview a couple of moving companies. One mover who didn't quote the lowest price had the best safety record with no claims by prior customers, so making that decision was easy. The difficulty now facing us was timing. How long would we be living in the apartment, unable to move our furniture and goods into the new Framingham house? What would we do with the furniture while we were in limbo? Put it in storage for an extra fee?

Fortunately, the moving company agreed to keep it on the truck.

My sister Sue returned with her husband, Fred, the weekend Charles and I moved into the apartment. We took only the clothes and items we needed for day-to-day living, as well as fragile items we didn't want the movers to touch. While Sue and I continued to pack and move these items, Fred entertained Charles in the new apartment.

Although I hid it well, I wavered on the brink of emotional collapse throughout these many false starts. I was totally exhausted. I just could not have handled one more thing. But though I didn't know how much I needed it initially, the support of so many caring people allowed my weakened and overwhelmed soul to hang on so I could continue on to the next challenge. I am certain now that it is only because of them that I survived that ordeal.

LOOKING FOR ANSWERS FROM HOLISTIC MEDICINE

Meanwhile, we weren't getting the kinds of answers we wanted from mainstream physicians, so we tried a holistic doctor.

The holistic doctor we selected was listed in a directory of "natural and holistic" practitioners we got from Sandi, a friend of ours who successfully fought breast cancer for a number of years. This doctor had a medical degree, but she also used alternative tests and procedures.

She took a careful history of Charles's health and health habits. After hearing his story, she prepared numerous tests for him to take at home—comprehensive digestive stool analysis, intestinal permeability, detoxification profile, and saliva and urine tests. She also took a blood test at the office. Surely one of these would show a cause for Charles's problem, we thought. Each test had complicated instructions with explicit actions to be taken within precise time frames. Then, adding to the complexity, they had specific instructions for how to pack and ship the specimens we collected.

One test required the collection of Charles's stool in a cup (not from the toilet) and mashing it to the consistency of soup. The saliva test had Charles take a NoDoz caplet at 9:00 AM, chew a cotton roll for forty-five seconds at 11:00 AM, and chew another cotton roll at 5:00 PM. He had to avoid caffeine for six hours with this test.

The urine test started with collecting a urine specimen in a small cup at 9:00 PM. Using a pipette, we had to transfer some of the urine from the cup into a tube. Before going to bed, Charles had to swallow two Tylenol and two Bayer aspirin tablets. For the next ten hours, until 7:00 AM, we collected every drop of urine.

Just doing *one* of these tests would have been difficult enough. But we did complete each one—I hope correctly. After all of these efforts, the doctor reviewed each of the results and still did not find a concrete alternative explanation for Charles's worsening symptoms. Frustrated and disappointed, we had no new cause or name for the condition Charles now lived with every day.

Caregiving Affirmation:
Be aware that you'll win some and lose some when
trying new medical treatments.

However, when she learned about Charles's limited nutrition habits—eating the same foods nearly every day—she recommended some vitamin and mineral pills. She had Charles begin taking green food supplements (GFSs), which she called "green food stuff"—capsules that contain dried leaves, sprouts, and vegetables. The GFSs proved extremely helpful later in the disease, helping him pass stools. We added coenzyme Q10 and ginkgo biloba, both of which she touted as being able to help with the memory and brain function he desperately wanted to retain.

Though we continued to order the GFSs and other pills, we stopped visiting this doctor when it was clear to her and us that she could find no new answers. Charles's baffling disease continued its game of hide-and-seek.

NEW HOPES

Charles lived in a progressively deteriorating body, so he clung to any glimmer of hope. And we did have some new hopes.

VOICE-ACTIVATED COMPUTER

Voice-activated software sounded like a great solution to Charles's deteriorating handwriting and dwindling ability to visually follow horizontal lines. His company offered to purchase and install it on his computer. In 1997 this technology was still very new, but the reviews sounded like it might actually work. All Charles would have to do was simply speak into the computer and let it do the typing, right?

Charles brought his laptop home, newly loaded with the software, and tried to make it work. We practiced together to help him memorize the official way to say the alphabet—alpha, bravo, Charlie, delta—in order to spell out words the computer didn't recognize. Then we tried using it.

Charles spoke into the computer: "Now is the time for all good men to come to the aid of their party." As I watched the screen, the computer typed only a few of the words correctly. In reading the instructions to see what to do next, we realized that the computer needed to "learn" Charles's pronunciation. He should speak each word slowly, watching to make sure that the computer typed in the correct word. If not, he had to retype the right word immediately, before saying the next one. That was how the computer would know which word to type the next time Charles said it.

As we practiced, Charles became more and more aggravated. I began to realize that he would not be able to use this software alone for quite some time, if ever. The main problem? He couldn't easily find and follow the words on the screen to know when the computer typed them incorrectly. Nonetheless, he struggled to make it succeed.

There had to be a way.

But as time went on, we realized that even with my help at home, the software needed a sighted person to make it work. The staff at Web couldn't spend the time Charles needed to get the computer comfortable with his pronunciations. If this technology was developed to help blind people, it had a long way to go! So much for the promise of voice activation. Another hope was shattered.

ACUPUNCTURE

"Do they hurt?" I asked about the needles the first time Charles tried acupuncture.

"No, they make me feel good," he replied.

But just getting a good feeling from the session was not enough. Charles hoped that Li Jung's magic—thin acupuncture needles placed in his head, neck, arms, torso, and legs—would do more. He hoped it would take away some of his body's severe stiffness and rigidity. He also hoped it would help alleviate the slight slurring of his speech that had been developing.

We trudged into Boston's Chinatown every Saturday. Li's clinic, located across the street from the St. Francis homeless shelter, had three small exam rooms, each with a long, thin table and extra chair. Li juggled clients simultaneously in all three rooms—inserting needles in one client, then, while that person relaxed with Chinese instrumental music playing in the background, setting up the next client.

In somewhat broken English, Li exuded great confidence in being able to help Charles. "I had success with similar problem in past. You should feel improvement soon." Then, Li—smaller than Charles—put one of his legs behind Charles's and in a flash had whipped him up onto the narrow table to begin his treatment.

After the first few visits, Charles said that he felt some improvement in his walking. But I wondered if that was the result of the acupuncture or just a placebo effect. Nonetheless, I encouraged him to believe that the acupuncture did help. We also began to notice that his speech stopped slurring and that the intermittent cough he had recently been experiencing went away.

It was hard to determine if the acupuncture or the new drug, Mirapex, caused his improvements. Because he started both of them at about the same time, it was impossible to know for sure. My skepticism, though, told me that the Mirapex probably had the greatest impact.

As time went on, Charles admitted in a disappointed voice, "I don't think it's helping anymore." Nonetheless, he continued the acupuncture treatments for almost a year. At the very minimum, they offered him a half hour to rest and feel good. And whether they were successful or not, Charles enjoyed the treat I gave him after every session. On the way home, I would double-park on Boylston Street and run inside Finagle a Bagel to get his favorite super cinnamon bagel—a doughy circular tube filled with raisins and covered with sugar crystals. His eyes would sparkle at the luscious taste as he bit into the bagel.

OTHER PROMISING THERAPIES

"Frozen shoulder," one doctor said, diagnosing the cause of Charles's pain. Lately Charles had been experiencing a significant ache in his shoulder, especially at night, ruining his already fitful sleep. "Here are some stretches and exercises you can do to help," he said as he gave us a handout with about seven different poses diagrammed on it. I'm sure they would have worked if Charles had stuck with them, but he didn't, and the pain got worse.

But physical therapy, for which Charles's primary care physician gave him a referral, *did* work. Though this was yet another thing to add to our hectic schedule, Charles saw Dawn at the physical therapy clinic twice a week, usually on Mondays and Wednesdays. Sometimes she would start with an ultrasound treatment, warming his muscles for the intense but slow stretching she would do. Other times, she would use a moist heating pad.

With Charles's muscles warmed, Dawn used her entire body weight to push against his inflexible muscles. Push and hold, push and hold. She spent a number of minutes working on each joint— doing not just his shoulders but also his hips. She remarked in astonishment, "I've never had a patient with muscles this stiff." In some odd way, that made Charles feel special and unique.

After she completed the session, she measured the progress. At first, Charles had pitiful flexibility, which caused the pain in his shoulder. Over several weeks of therapy, Dawn increased the distance each joint could move and eventually eliminated the shoulder pain. When Charles's series of visits ended, she instructed us to continue the stretching at home, and this time we did.

Along with the physical therapy referral, his doctor also authorized occupational and speech therapy.

The speech therapist found working with Charles totally overwhelming. All of her exercises required that Charles read the words on her practice sheet. Because she was visibly flustered and unable to accommodate his needs, our first appointment with her was our last.

We didn't have much better success with the occupational therapist, although he kept trying diligently to make a difference. He made a splint for Charles's right hand to help keep the disease from contracting his fingers into a fist. He also attempted techniques to help Charles with activities to better manage at work, such as with dialing the phone and using the computer. But Charles's condition would just not oblige, rendering most of the exercises and techniques useless.

In addition to therapies for his body, physicians and friends encouraged Charles to get counseling. This was not a foreign concept to him, as he spent years in therapy with a psychologist after the breakup of his first marriage. But that particular counselor would have retired by now, he suspected.

I called Blue Cross Blue Shield's Employee Assistance Program (EAP) to see if anyone there could recommend someone who had experience counseling people with degenerative diseases. Of the three counselors recommended, two could not see us in the evenings or on weekends. That left only one. He practiced in our city and assured us that he had experience counseling groups of people with various medical conditions.

Charles and I went together for a few sessions—just long enough for us to realize that the counselor didn't ask good questions or facilitate our conversation. Charles and I had enough savvy in this area to carry on our own discussion; we didn't need to pay a therapist for that. So we stopped going.

Then Tom, the EAP director contracted with Web Industries, called and invited us to have a session with him. At that first visit, we recognized the value Tom would bring to our issues. Looking like a counselor with his handlebar mustache and corduroy jacket, Tom asked in his gentle voice, "Tell me, Charles, what causes you frustration." After listening to Charles's response, he slowly asked probing questions to move Charles along in his ability to cope.

During one session, he gave Charles a handout titled "Dream Sheet." It listed items such as *travel, money, family, education,* and *activities.* Tom said to Charles, "I'd like you to take this home and think about which of these are most important for you now. Then circle the ones that you would like to focus on in light of your disease's progression. Jot down the ways that you'll accomplish these. We'll talk about this at our next session."

When we got home, we noticed the instructions indicated that after Charles circled the activities and listed how he would do them, he should set the Dream Sheet aside for twenty-four hours. When coming back to it, he should write down the "why" for each circled item. The instructions said that if he couldn't articulate a one-sentence reason for that activity, it was not important enough to stay on the list.

Charles circled eight items. Under the first one he circled, *activities,* he noted that he would do an e-mail thought for the day to his colleagues and workers. His reason why—to stay in touch. He circled *shared time* and added *with Janet.* He circled *friendship* and noted that he'd like to continue having friends over every so often, to stay in touch. He selected *the helping of others* and mentioned delivering doughnuts to the workers at the Framingham plant to show his support for them. Meeting with a pastor and meditating on scriptures would help him rethink his faith and deal with the items *religious study* and *your mind.* He circled *respect* but didn't provide an activity or a "why" for that one. Finally, he chose *reading,* noting that he wanted to have books read to him that would give him energy and from which he could learn.

He noted an overall "why" on the sheet as well: to "learn how to have fun, and to continue and add to the things I enjoy."

Another exercise that Tom assigned required Charles to evaluate himself in several areas, including *appearance, family, financial, social, spiritual, mental,* and *career.* Charles rated himself "excellent" (a 5 on a five-point scale) on making sure he got medical checkups; on nutrition; on having a forgiving attitude; on being supportive of others, respectful, caring, and loving; on his sense of purpose and imagination; on continuing his education; and on his level of curiosity. Most telling, though, were the things he rated a 2 or 3: exercise program, listening habits, sense of humor, self-confidence, inner peace, prayer, religious study, and belief in God. These lower ratings prompted him to think of actions he could take, including doing range-of-motion exercises once a day; using listening skills when listening to me; having a fun day every Friday with a special lunch, frozen yogurt, and a movie; trying to maintain the best in himself to build his self-confidence; and looking for solutions for his lack of inner peace.

These exercises helped him focus on what he could still do instead of dwelling on what he could no longer do. And though he'd continue to struggle with accepting this disease, they allowed him to realize that his life could still have purpose.

The sessions with Tom also helped me.

Charles vented his anger with the ways I bugged him. I think Charles was beginning to see me as the bad guy because of things like insisting that he wear a pad for his bladder-control problem and warning him, for his own safety, not to try things his body could no longer do.

I realized through this process, and through earlier events, that I tend in some ways to be more like a man, as John Gray describes in his popular book *Men Are from Mars, Women Are from Venus.* His theory is that men tend to want to solve the issues women discuss with them, instead of just listening with empathy the way women tend to do. I'm a solver. My first instinct, no matter how hard I try to curb it, is to solve. Give me a problem, and I'll quickly come up with a number of plausible resolutions.

Throughout Charles's disease, I'm sure I tended to be both the cheerleader and solution finder. At times, that served us both well. But at other times, I'm sure Charles needed only an empathetic ear—without any of the solutions. And that was hard for me.

I'm not sure, even after those counseling sessions, that I became effective at eliminating the source of Charles's accusations. And most of the time I accepted that I was simply the object of his frustrations. But it hurt me deeply to see how this disease had dampened our wonderfully congenial relationship.

Caregiving Affirmation:
You don't always have to be a fixer. Sometimes
your loved one needs only your empathy.

First Experience with a PSP Support Group

"This is Ellen Katz," the woman said after I picked up the phone at work. "I'm the executive director of the Society for PSP [Progressive Supranuclear Palsy]. I'm coming to Boston for a neurological convention, and I wondered if you thought we could have a support group meeting with caregivers and people with PSP in the Boston area." I had volunteered as a contact person when I joined the society, which was how Ellen got my name.

"We'd love that," I replied, encouraged by the thought that we might actually meet someone else with PSP.

I coordinated the meeting at my workplace, Blue Cross Blue Shield of Massachusetts, in downtown Boston. About ten people attended along with Charles and me. Unfortunately, none actually had PSP except Charles. All were family members or friends of a person with PSP. As we circled the room discussing our connection with PSP, the caregivers shared what PSP had done to their loved ones and what they found had worked best in caring for them.

One person mentioned that a Hoyer patient lift made it easy for her to move her husband, who could no longer walk, from one place to another, such as from bed and into a wheelchair. Another talked about the best kind of wheelchairs and must-have attachments she'd bought. Two twin daughters described a system they used to help communicate with their mother, who could barely talk because of slurring her words. One finger up meant *yes* and two meant *no.* A husband mentioned some sort of stuff to put into liquids to keep his wife from choking. Another mentioned the difficult decision of installing a feeding tube. They talked about the doctors to whom they had taken their loved ones—all the same doctors Charles and I had visited.

The more they talked, the more depressed I got, and worried about how Charles would react to hearing about all this. He could still walk, but he needed assistance. He could still talk. He could still swallow. For these caregivers' loved ones, the PSP was much more advanced. Would Charles get to that same place someday? What was he thinking about the gloomy conversation?

Charles didn't say much during the meeting. Bracing myself to lift up his spirits, I asked on our way home, "What did you think about the meeting tonight?" To my surprise, he simply replied, "It made me feel normal to know about others with PSP. I'm not alone."

Our connection to the Society of PSP led us to attend its biannual symposium in Baltimore. During the one-day program, we heard from the leading researchers in the field of PSP. They told which medications had promise and which appeared to not work. They described the physiology of the disease process. They mentioned items and tips that would help with day-to-day living, such as using walkers weighted in the front and raising a plate of food with a couple of phone books to make it easier to get food to the mouth.

Once again, Charles was comforted by being with people who struggled like him to make it through this dark tunnel of a disease as gracefully as possible.

Caregiving Affirmation:
Be aware that your perspective may be
very different from your loved one's.

GUINEA PIG FOR POSITRON EMISSION TOMOGRAPHY SCANS
"It takes a picture of the functioning of the brain," Charles's neurologist from a prominent Boston hospital said, explaining the work-

ings of the positron emission tomography (PET) scan he ordered for
Charles. "It's different from MRI [magnetic resonance imaging],
which is a two-dimensional x-ray. The PET scan is like a three-
dimensional picture, showing what is actually happening with the
functioning of the brain." He then went on to say, "We'll need to
enroll Charles into a study in order for him to get the test."

Convinced that this new technology might actually find out where
his brain was malfunctioning, Charles agreed to take part in the
study.

The teaching hospitals in Boston often acquire experimental tech-
nologies before others do. In 1997 this prominent hospital had one
of the early PET scan machines. However, we didn't understand how
new and therefore unpredictable it really was, and I'm not sure the
hospital did either.

The morning of the scheduled test, we wandered the labyrinth of
hallways to find the neurological radiology lab. Once we arrived at
what appeared to be the check-in desk, the receptionist greeted us
and said the test would take a good part of the day. They agreed to
take care of Charles and instructed me to come back later that afternoon to pick him up.

When I returned to the lab, I found Charles sitting alone in the
waiting room. He said that they couldn't perform the test—something
about the machine not working. I asked, "Did you get any lunch?"

"No," he said. "They only got me a soda."

Though Charles didn't seem fazed by this, I seethed as I thought
of him sitting in the waiting room all day with nothing to eat—and
nothing to do. He couldn't even read the magazines. I was perturbed,
but we desperately wanted to have this test done and find out the
results. So we rescheduled for another day.

This time, the receptionist called the morning before we left and
said they couldn't get the machine or isotope to work again. We
scheduled a new appointment.

Finally Charles actually had the test. I stayed with him that time.
They injected a radioactive isotope into his arm and then waited for
it to circulate throughout his body—and into his brain. Then they
laid him on a table and placed a warm, pliable sheet of plaster over

his face, with eyes, mouth, and nose cut out, allowing it to form to his face's shape. This, they said, would keep his head from moving while the machine meticulously scanned his brain, section by section. Charles willingly obeyed all of their instructions, keeping perfectly still during the test.

It took a number of weeks after the test for the researcher to get the results to Charles's neurologist. When we finally met with him, he said, "Your results are markedly abnormal. It appears that your brain has plenty of dopamine, which is unusual for the Parkinson-plus diseases. But it doesn't look like the dopamine is getting into the brain cells." Then the neurologist suggested we do a follow-up test to study this mystery further. "It will look at the dopamine receptor sites," he explained.

Again we had starts and stops in actually getting this second test done, as the lab struggled with the temperamental machine and isotopes. But once Charles had the test, the neurologist was puzzled by the results, saying they were unremarkable. He agreed with Charles and me that taking the results of the first and second test with us for our appointment at the U.S. government's National Institutes of Health (NIH) would be the best next step. Meanwhile, he would talk to the other neurologists at his hospital to see if Charles's symptoms and PET scan results could help diagnose his condition.

We wondered whether the people at the hospital really cared about Charles as a person, or whether they were more interested in just studying his puzzling disease.

A BIRTHDAY AT THE NATIONAL INSTITUTES OF HEALTH

What a way to celebrate a birthday! Charles spent his forty-eighth birthday, October 14, 1997, undergoing neurological exams at the NIH.

Charles's neurologist from Boston Medical Center requested and received approval for our visit to the NIH. Our federal tax dollars were at work—the NIH funded the testing. But we had to pay all other expenses. We kept them down by taking advantage of the special NIH patient rate at the Park Inn International Hotel and driving from Boston to Washington rather than flying, even though it took us eight hours.

To pass the time during our travel, I played cassette tapes of *Chicken Soup for the Soul,* and we listened to the short stories of inspiration. After every vignette, I tried to prompt a discussion on what we had learned from it, hoping these would lift his spirits. In doing so, though, I realized that Charles didn't seem to be able to clearly follow the stories.

But my biggest struggle with our travel came when a restroom wasn't handy at the time Charles needed it. So I pulled the car over to the side of the road and used an open car door to give Charles privacy, helping him stand and urinate into a plastic container.

In preparation for the visit, I had helped Charles complete the seven-page neuromedical history. It asked if any family members had neurological conditions and if Charles's mother had had any difficulties with his birth or with Charles during his early childhood. We had to record Charles's exposure to chemicals and past surgeries. It asked us to describe any symptoms he had experienced, listing things like depression, failing memory, speech or visual issues, problems with walking and balance, and clumsiness with the hands. And of course, they wanted to know all of the medications he was taking or had taken. Once again, our symptom sheet was helpful.

Armed with this report, as well as copies of Charles's medical records and PET scan films, we drove around the wandering campus of the NIH in Bethesda, Maryland, to find the clinical center where various MDs and PhDs were to perform three days' worth of tests.

Charles couldn't even properly sign the admission forms, which required his signature in several spots. He hadn't attempted to sign his name in quite some time. The best he could do was to squiggle the pen around when I positioned his hand at each signature line. No two signatures turned out alike, or even vaguely resembled his name. That made him feel that he had failed his first task at the NIH—and the testing hadn't even officially started.

On the first day, we met with the primary neurologist. She examined Charles for over an hour, pushing him to see if he could hold his balance, which he couldn't, checking his reflexes and sensory perceptions, and conducting basic visual tests. She finally said in a caring voice, "I suspect that Charles has CBGD. But we'll need to see how the other tests turn out to rule out other potential diagnoses." That was not what we wanted to hear. CBGD is even worse than PSP, affecting more areas of the brain and, in turn, the body, and carried an even shorter life expectancy. Charles, however, seemed indifferent to her comments.

That afternoon, the neuro-ophthalmologist tested Charles's syncopated eye movements. He told us, "Charles's visual attention is shot. While his reflexes are okay, he appears to have apraxia of the saccades—that's when the eyes forget how to do something." He went on to say that the deterioration must be in the left side of the brain, mostly affecting his right eye's vision. He then used a term that one of our Boston neurologists had mentioned—Balint syndrome. "This explains Charles's difficulty in controlling where to look and his trouble fixating on objects," the doctor explained. But he didn't think that Charles's complex pattern of problems necessarily meant CBGD, which raised our hopes.

We spent three grueling days going from one lab to the next. There, health-care practitioners laid Charles on a radiology table for an MRI, drew blood for genetic testing, gave him speech and swallowing tests, and ended with a neuropsychology exam.

I was mesmerized as I watched Charles take the swallowing test. The technicians gave him foods of different consistencies and watched on the x-ray screen as he swallowed each one. We could all easily see why Charles had been coughing when swallowing water or juice. Liquids clearly got stuck in a pouch on the way through, triggering his need to cough. Only swallowing a second time could get it all down. We used that helpful knowledge when we went home. Every time Charles coughed while eating or drinking, I'd say, "Try to swallow again." And it worked.

The speech therapist also shed some light on several peculiar things I had observed recently. The first she called perseveration. I noticed it when Charles and I performed speech exercises on our morning runs. Every time I gave Charles a word with which to build a sentence, he got stuck in a rut of always using the word process. For example, if I gave him the word meeting, he'd put it in a sentence like, "We talked about the process at the meeting." Or if I gave him the word *maintain*, he'd say something like, "They maintained the *process*." Once he started using the word *process*, he couldn't create a sentence without it. The speech therapist instructed us that the way to get him out of that groove was to distract him and do something totally different. But once we got home, I found that this advice was not easy to implement.

"Name as many animals as you can," the therapist said, getting ready to time Charles's response. She hit the stopwatch button. Charles said nothing. He couldn't think of any animal names. She then prompted, "They can be wild or domestic." By the end of the generous amount of time allotted, Charles had named only three kinds of animals—lions, tigers, and dogs. Next, the therapist took a number of objects out of her black bag one by one. Because of Charles's visual problems, she allowed him not only to look at them but also to feel each object. She simply asked him to name each item—hammer, thumbtack, nail clippers, and so forth. To my astonishment, he couldn't do it.

The speech therapist said this was caused by aphasia. Charles couldn't retrieve the words he wanted, or he would say the opposite of what he meant to say. This explained what I had been noticing lately, with Charles saying yes when he meant to say no, and vice versa. The therapist suggested that we ask more clarifying questions to pull the right words out of him. "Be patient and don't get discouraged," she urged.

In the last session of the three days, a neuropsychologist gave Charles an apraxia test. Another peculiarity of Charles's disease, apraxia didn't allow him to make the deliberate movements he wanted to make. He couldn't clap his hands if he wanted to, or purposely snap his fingers. Though this feature was seemingly harmless at this stage of the disease, it became a huge problem when Charles could no longer talk. How would he be able to make people—including those closest to him—understand him?

The results of test after test highlighted the tremendous changes in Charles's physical and mental capabilities. I didn't directly ask Charles how he felt about the experience, because I was afraid to highlight his losses. And I wondered if he even realized the over-whelming way that he failed each test. For me, however, a new understanding about this strange disease emerged, and I learned tips for dealing with it. Also, hearing that the unusual symptoms Charles lived with each day actually had names helped to validate the things I had been noticing. This gave me a sense of comfort—I hadn't been imagining things.

We had both hoped that Charles's condition would be definitively diagnosed and that there might be new treatments available from the best experts in the nation. But even though the report we later received suggested that he might have CBGD, questions still remained—meaning that Charles would have to undergo more tests when we were back in Boston. With so much anticipation, and then the actual testing, I don't even remember if we actually celebrated Charles's birthday.

Caregiving Affirmation:
Because doctors are constantly making new discoveries,
consider taking a trip to the National Institutes of Health.

SEEING THROUGH HEARING

When I met Charles, I quickly learned that he went to see just about every movie that came out. Going to the movies was his way of occupying the lonely time after he and his first wife separated. We weren't that diligent about getting to every movie, but after we married, movies still played a big part in our entertainment and release from the tensions of the work week.

A year earlier, in 1996, I'd realized that Charles couldn't follow the action in fast-paced movies. When we walked out of the theater after seeing the first *Mission: Impossible* movie, Charles admitted, "The people on the screen moved too fast. I couldn't keep up with them."

Then as time passed, I wondered whether, with his shrinking peripheral vision, he could even catch the drama taking place in other types of movies. One of the pleasures he'd enjoyed on an almost weekly basis seemed to be slipping away. But our hopes rose when a local theater advertised a new audiotape system for their visually impaired patrons. It was first put to use when *Titanic* came out, so we gave it a try.

We picked up the headset and tape player from the customer service desk and then took our seat in the large theater. Once we set things up, Charles sat peacefully for about the first ten minutes of *Titanic*.

Then I noticed him starting to get uneasy and squirm a bit. I asked, "How is it working? Can you follow the story?"

"No," he grumbled.

"Can I listen for a minute to see what it's doing?" I whispered. I put the headphones on and listened as the narrator, between bits of dialogue in the movie, described in detail the scene on the boat and the background action—such as how the dining room was set up and the waiter walking over to the table. "Charles, is this too complicated for you to follow?" I asked.

"Yes," he replied in disappointment.

I think the disease had hampered his ability to process a lot of information as quickly as he once had. With no other ideas, I simply put the headphones back on Charles and suggested, "Do the best you can. I don't know what else to try."

While I became totally engrossed in the movie, Charles continued to fidget and missed the impact of the film—effectively marking the end of his ability to enjoy the big screen.

Caregiving Affirmation:
Accept that you won't be able to fix everything;
even creative solutions will sometimes fail.

FINDING THE GIFTS

TRIBUTES PROVIDE ENCOURAGEMENT

People often debate over which kind of death they might prefer—dying suddenly, as from a massive heart attack, or slowly, from a degenerative condition.

From the perspective of caregiver, I prefer a slower death. With Charles, it gave me millions of opportunities to provide support and love. In the midst of the tragedy, I found it rewarding to let him know frequently the value he had brought to my life.

I'm not sure that Charles would have agreed that a slower death was better, as he was the one suffering all the losses. But because people knew Charles was dying, they, too, had a chance—one they often took advantage of—to share with him what he had meant to them. Many found it difficult to talk to him in person about such deep feelings, so they wrote down their thoughts. This may have also allowed them to come to grips with Charles's terminal illness.

Lauren, a Web Industries employee who professed that Charles was her mentor, knew how much he had touched people at work and beyond. Not telling us, Lauren asked these people to write to him, and forty-five responded. Lauren then typed up each of these responses and had them bound into a booklet that she presented to Charles. And because he could no longer read, she also dictated them onto cassette tapes.

The tributes shared phenomenal stories, from factory workers to CEOs, about how Charles had nurtured their needs, given them wisdom, made them feel valued, and changed their lives. They had learned from Charles how to care about others as well as to see the best in themselves, treat themselves with respect, and give themselves grace. They also told of Charles's influence in teaching them how important it is to listen, how to be committed to the potential of each individual, to not give up on people, and to be dedicated to always learning. And they demonstrated how he had given them the confidence to believe they could make a difference.

In short, Charles had helped each of them be a better person.

When Charles first heard these tributes, he couldn't believe that people really felt that way about him. Despite his tremendous humility, these tributes lifted his slumping spirits many times throughout the final years of his illness. They provided him with a living eulogy. Listening to them, especially at night when he couldn't sleep, revealed to his doubting self that he truly *had* impacted these people's lives.

Charles would have missed this opportunity if he had died suddenly instead of slowly. Without the tragic circumstance of this neurological condition, when would these people have given Charles these accolades?

During Charles's illness, periodically we pulled out the over-stuffed, tattered bag filled with a stash of letters. He'd received the letters in September 1995, when, at the point where symptoms of his disease first appeared, he'd attended the Christian men's retreat I mentioned in the previous chapter. After he returned home, Charles had told me, in tears, how special those letters were to him, and that he was not worthy of the wonderful things that people expressed. Now, during his fight with this neurological disease, these letters provided concrete emotional support.

Charles also found encouragement in the many e-mails and occasional calls and letters that people used to express their thoughts. When an especially touching e-mail arrived, I'd print it out and read it to Charles whenever depression hit him. While these helped Charles, I, too, was blessed by being able to share them with him.

I felt the full weight of the contrast between a slow versus a sudden death when nearly a year after Charles died, I attended the wedding of Patty, one of my staff members. As with most brides, Patty's smile and beauty radiated throughout the wedding and reception. It was a special moment when Maco, Patty's new husband, shared a touching story about how he'd dreamed of marrying Patty before they were even dating, and then how he passionately pursued her. His awe and love for her overflowed from his words.

But at the end of the evening, during the partying, Maco's trim and fit brother-in-law, David, died on the dance floor of a massive heart attack. No one—not even David—had known that he had any heart problems. He was only fifty years old. Patty's parents shared with me what they had learned at the funeral—that David was a devoted family man, in the midst of a successful career. Unfortunately, though, I doubt that he had the rich opportunity that Charles did, to hear the many tributes of his legacy.

PULLING THE FAMILY TOGETHER

"I don't need anything," I'd reply when someone in my family or Charles's would ask how to help. And I truly didn't believe they could offer any meaningful assistance. None of them lived near the Boston area. The next closest relative lived in West Virginia, with others in Illinois, Arkansas, Georgia, and Florida.

"Well, I'm coming in two weeks to spend the weekend," one of my sisters insisted. Though I still didn't understand what she might do to help, I responded, "Okay, if you really want to. But I don't think there's anything special you can do."

My family members had helped tremendously during our move, but now that we were settled, I couldn't imagine what else they might do. In the ensuing months, however, I learned how wrong I was. It wasn't until they started to visit that I realized how much help I needed, and the unique skills that each one could bring. And I was totally astonished to learn that every month, my four sisters and brother each contributed thirty dollars to a fund that sent one of them, or my mother, to visit about once every six weeks or so.

My sister Barb helped with my mounting stack of bills. She organized them, wrote the necessary checks, mailed the payments, and tossed the junk mail. Her husband, Jack, spent hours on the phone calling various resources and his company's EAP to get lists of agencies that could provide home health aides and other assistance I would surely need in the future.

My sister Sue always found heavy-duty cleaning projects to keep her busy when she visited. She shampooed rugs, cleaned the floors, and whirled through the entire house with her cleaning supplies. Sue also timed a visit in 1998 with her daughter Rachel to help me with the neighborhood party for thirty-five people that I had planned at our new home. I had underestimated the effort it would take to prepare for the party and also host it, as Charles required full-time attention throughout the event. Sue and Rachel kept preparing and replenishing the food trays, filling beverage glasses, and handling the myriad issues that arose while Charles and I simply greeted the guests.

On his visits, my brother Doug, with tools in hand, helped get the little nagging things completed around the house that I'm useless at doing.

Later in the disease, my sister Lois, who left her five children and husband at their home in Florida, spent hours helping me set up a federal tax ID, fill out unemployment and worker's compensation insurance forms, and prepare the special federal tax forms for the aides we eventually needed to hire after Charles had stopped working and stayed at home. She also helped me organize Charles's medical and dependent-care expenses to maximize the deductions for our income tax return. As you can imagine, the government doesn't make this process easy. I absolutely couldn't have figured out all of this on my own, let alone had the time to do it.

My sister Carolyn helped from her home in Florida by calling all the references for the aides we interviewed and giving me a report of her findings. When she visited, leaving her husband Tony with their two young children, she spent hours in the kitchen cooking meals and baking desserts that she loaded into the freezer for us to eat once she left.

My mother visited the most frequently, doing motherly tasks—laundry, cleaning, cooking, rearranging, shopping, and errands. She even helped with hiring the aides we would soon need.

In contrast, Charles hadn't seemed close to his family in all the years we'd been together. He hadn't even encouraged them to attend our wedding, so none of them did. Charles visited his family only occasionally. His parents seemed awkward in social settings, a source of embarrassment for him since childhood. I understand that at dinnertime when Charles and his two younger brothers were growing up, his parents would play chess at one end of the table with the boys quietly eating at the other. Before Charles's illness, we coordinated a couple of small reunions at his parents' home in Arkansas to begin to build a sense of family. His illness helped crystallize the growing connection.

Because by this point Charles's mother had Alzheimer's disease and his father had Parkinson's disease, they couldn't be actively involved in assisting us. But his brother Ken regularly stayed in touch, calling every weekend. What a change from our former relationship with him—Charles might have talked to him only a dozen times during our first fifteen years of marriage. Ken also traveled to visit us a few times. Because he's extraordinarily handy, I always had ready for him a list of heavy-duty fixes that I needed made around the house—such as stabilizing the wooden steps off our back deck.

Even his wife, Shari, who also visited periodically, swung a hammer effectively. Ken still remarks when he calls me each week, "One of the blessings of Charles's illness was discovering in you the sister I never had."

David, Charles's other brother, made a point to visit a few times with his wife, Jayne, and their younger children. He wanted them to know Charles before it was too late. Because of the kids, David and Jayne couldn't help around the house, but they allowed Charles and me to do fun things with the kids, which gave us both lots of enjoyment.

Engrossed in our own lives over the years, Charles and I had unfortunately missed various family events when they didn't fit into our schedule. In a way, I'm grateful that Charles and I were the first among our family members to have a significant medical crisis, because that gave me the chance to see how family can really respond and help. If one of our family members had been the first with such needs, I'm not certain I would have been as supportive as they were to us. I'm sure I would have called to check in every now and then. But I imagine that I would have felt that my life was too busy and my work too important to make the effort to visit or help in more substantial ways.

Thankfully, I learned, through our experience, the sacrifices that make family relationships so valuable. And I hope I will live up to the challenge when the opportunity to give comes my way.

Caregiving Affirmation:
Look for the gifts that only this type of tragedy affords.

OTHERS GIVE BEYOND OUR EXPECTATIONS

The best of human nature reveals itself during difficult times, as U.S. citizens witnessed after September 11, 2001. I had the good fortune of experiencing the wonders of the human spirit during Charles's illness. Charles's friends seemed to know the best ways to meet his needs.

Loren, a friend from the ESOP Association, understood how important books were to Charles. And he knew that Charles's eyes could no longer manage the task of moving across the page to follow the unfolding words. Charles now needed someone to read to him. Books on tape provided one avenue for addressing that need. But many of the books that interested Charles had not been put on tape.

One day when Loren visited, he brought a stack of eight cassette tapes held together with a thick rubber band. He had coordinated the efforts of six of Charles's friends from around the country to each record a chapter or two on tape. Loren had bought the book, ripped it apart into chapters, sent the chapters and a blank cassette tape to each person among the network of volunteers, and followed up with everyone to ensure that he received all the recorded tapes.

After the surprise of this first delivery, Loren then asked Charles what other books he'd like to have on tape. Over the next few years, Loren coordinated a growing team of recording volunteers that also included people from my staff, reading books such as *Tuesdays with Morrie, God and the Philosophers: The Reconciliation of Faith and Reason, The Living Company, The Path to Love: Spiritual Strategies for Healing, Leading Without Power: Finding Hope in Serving Community,* and *Leading Minds: An Anatomy of Leadership.*

Charles enjoyed not only hearing the books but also remembering his friends as he recognized their voices on the tape. It didn't matter at all that they didn't have professional recording voices.

Loren also coordinated another thoughtful gift. Charles's employee ownership friends recognized the importance of his daily jogs, and they also knew the challenge of running in New England weather. They planned to give him a treadmill.

I knew about the surprise in advance. I invited Loren and a handful of friends from the local employee ownership community to have dinner with us. While we ate dinner in one part of the house, others brought the treadmill in through another part and placed it in one of the spare bedrooms.

After dinner, they explained that they had something to show Charles and took him to the bedroom where the treadmill was. I could sense the tenderness between Charles and his friends. They assisted him onto the treadmill and had him take a test run, someone holding each of his arms. Their kindness overwhelmed Charles.

He had always been the one who gave to others, so he found it difficult to receive. I'm sure that even as wonderful as it was to receive
these gifts and kindnesses, a part of him struggled because he
couldn't give back in the same way.

Nonetheless, he recognized that the compassion shown during
his illness went beyond friends and family. "Even strangers in air-
ports help me," Charles constantly remarked in amazement. With
his continued travel, he experienced airline personnel graciously
lifting him onto the aisle wheelchair that easily rolled him to his
seat, or assisting him onto the motorized cart to make his connections. At every turn, people everywhere offered to help, even with
little things like holding open the doors.

I, too, experienced wonderful kindnesses, not only from my
friends but also from my colleagues and staff members. My various
leaders at Blue Cross Blue Shield went out of their way to make me
feel comfortable with juggling the demands of caregiving and working full-time. They understood my need to take Charles to his doctor visits, which were often lengthy; and as the disease progressed
over the next few years and Charles was now spending his days at
home, they also understood when I needed to stay home because
Charles's aide was ill.

My staff members took on more than their share, helping accomplish tasks that I would have normally done. In retrospect, I'm sure
that it allowed them to grow in more ways than even they expected.
But I would have been snowed under and paralyzed without their
willingness to help.

All that benevolence was proof that in a crisis, people are at their
finest. And then there was Cal.

CAL GIVES BACK
When in doubt about the inherent worth of people, something
that Charles so strongly believed in, I think of Cal.

With Charles's vision continuing to deteriorate, Cal started to visit
weekly to read to Charles. A machine operator who Charles had
mentored at the Web plant in Framingham, and an avid reader himself, Cal knew how Charles felt about books and learning new ideas.

During his weekly visits, Cal had quickly learned that I had no talent for cooking. Heating up frozen dinners is the extent of my ability. As time went on, he offered to cook for us one evening—and that turned into a long-standing tradition.

Every Tuesday when Cal visited, he put one of our royal blue barbecue aprons on his tall, fit body and began stirring up his now famous dishes—rice and beans or pasta with beans. And he used only all-natural ingredients—one requirement Cal followed religiously. I especially enjoyed walking into the house after a long day at work and taking in the wonderful smells of the spices and ingredients cooking together. In addition to feeding us, he also kept us entertained with his passionate discussions of world news.

But I understand from Cal and others that he didn't always have this giving nature. Cal had started working at Web's Framingham plant a few years earlier. Web had hired Cal when he had nowhere else to turn—because, as Cal explained, his alcoholism had ruled his life, causing him to lose his previous jobs.

Alcohol-free by the time he got the job at Web, Cal had the new start he needed. But at the time, it was just a job for Cal—until Charles happened in one Saturday afternoon, before symptoms of his illness had begun to appear. As vice president of manufacturing, he periodically visited the Framingham plant on the weekends to encourage the people working that extra day of the week.

On that Saturday, he saw Cal running one of the slitting machines and started up a conversation. Charles shared his passion for employee ownership with Cal, and tried to get him excited about the concept. I understand that at first, Cal resisted. Cal said to Charles, "Are you serious about this? I'm fifty years old now and don't have many chances left in life." Cal's cynical nature led him to think that employee ownership was just a scam to trick workers into getting more involved in their jobs.

But Charles must have convinced Cal that he was serious. Cal began to work with Charles as a spokesperson for employee ownership, appearing at conferences and leadership training programs. He became an example of the influence one person can have on another if that person truly believes in him.

Charles's terrible disease gave Cal an opportunity to give back to Charles. He consistently visited and cooked for us until Charles died. Even now, after Charles's death, he continues to cook at my house every few weeks. I take that opportunity to invite people important to Cal and to me—especially those who had a connection with Charles.

I've watched Cal continue to demonstrate Charles's influence on his life, especially with the friendships he's made on his numerous trips to Russia. One of the paradoxes of this dreadful disease is that it offered Cal the opportunity to give back in ways that not only encouraged Charles and me, but also helped Cal realize his own accomplishments and the personal growth he's achieved. Seeing the demonstration of that growth created another opportunity for me to find meaning in Charles's disease.

LEARNING IMPORTANT LIFE LESSONS

MESSAGES IN EASTERN TEACHINGS

Michael, Charles's friend through the employee ownership community and a reflective thinker, frequently donated books for me to read to Charles, or cassette tapes on Eastern philosophies for Charles to listen to. He felt that one author, Thich Nhat Hanh, provided especially helpful thoughts for Charles to consider in facing this illness. I began reading Hanh's book *Touching Peace: Practicing the Art of Mindful Living* out loud to Charles. About that same time, we also started reading *Wherever You Go There You Are: Mindfulness Meditation in Everyday Life,* by Jon Kabat-Zinn. Both books emphasize an important life concept of "being, not doing."

The books prompted many discussions between Charles and me. Both of us found our identities through the things we'd done. Neither of us felt comfortable with just being. Taking away his ability to do, the disease had now destroyed Charles's view of identity and worth in life—producing frustration and depression. He struggled hard to absorb that he was not what he *did* but *who* he was. Reading these books at least forced this concept into our consciousness, even though we might not have been able to fully apply it in our lives. We found it hard to break the American cultural emphasis we'd grown up with, which always seemed to first ask, "What do you *do?*"

In addition to instructing us in this new way of looking at ourselves, these books also taught the concept of being in the moment and truly being *present.* Looking ahead to where this disease would take Charles was very scary. If we could be in the moment, though, the future wouldn't loom so strongly, like a dark vacuum, sucking Charles's life away. Instead, we would appreciate what today had in store for us.

Taking it all one step further, these books encouraged us to make each moment count. I tried to use this simple notion to keep Charles focused, as best he could, on finding ways to capitalize on what he could do that day. This disease gave no promise of what tomorrow would bring.

Though we constantly struggled to apply them to our lives, the teachings were true. We could actually "touch peace" when we were mindful of these concepts.

FINDING HUMOR

"Stop and plop!" my brother-in-law Fred said just after he turned Charles to place him in front of the upholstered chair in our temporary apartment. Then Fred, who stood six foot four, assisted as Charles dropped his five feet six inches comfortably into place. Charles didn't have the coordination to slowly lower himself into the chair—he actually did plop into it.

Fred had to use that phrase only once for Charles to quickly adopt it. I always got a chuckle when Charles giggled and cheerily said, "Stop and plop!" every time I or someone else helped lower him into a chair.

On other occasions, he would break into a song triggered by something that was said. "Stand up," I'd say while assisting him during his morning shower. He'd stand up from his shower chair, soaking wet, and sing, "Stand up, stand up for Jesus, ye soldiers of the cross . . ." Once this pattern started, I could count on hearing him sing that old church hymn absolutely every morning.

Other commands would also trigger a song, but he didn't always get the words exactly right. When we jogged together, I'd instruct him that we needed to go "over there," to cross the street to get home. As soon as he heard those words, he'd start singing, "Over hill, over dale, we will hit the dusty trail . . . with a knickknack paddy-whack, give a dog a bone, this old man came rolling home." It didn't matter that he put two songs together, thinking they were one—he always sang those same words after my trigger of "over there."

And female nurses responded affectionately when Charles would start singing the Beatles' tune "I Want to Hold Your Hand" every time they grabbed his hand to take his blood pressure or assist him in some way.

Though Charles wasn't typically a spontaneous singer, he did have a reputation of being a prankster. I saw this side of him at family weddings. During my sister Barb's wedding reception in 1986, he instigated a plan and pulled the rest of us into it. He found Barb's honeymoon luggage, neatly packed in the back of my dad's white Lincoln Continental. In addition to sprinkling confetti throughout the luggage, he decided it would be very funny to take all of Barb's underwear. She would arrive in Hawaii and find that the only bra and panties that she had were the ones she was wearing—and in place of the missing underwear would be a note that read "We got you!"

Such a joke would be funny to most potential targets, who would probably just go out and buy some new underwear upon arriving at their destination. But as word of what we'd done reached my mother, aunt, and grandmother, they chided us that Barb was not the appropriate target for this prank. They said that Barb, who was well endowed, spent many frustrating hours shopping, trying to find bras that would fit. It wouldn't be easy for her to find replacements in Hawaii. "You've gone too far on this one," they said.

We finally persuaded Charles, the ringleader, that we had to amend our prank. We desperately tried to figure out how to make contact with Barb and Jack before they caught their plane. We couldn't do so in time—but after all our concern, Barb took the joke the way we had hoped. All was well.

When we were dating, Charles told me about the practical jokes he had initiated during college. The pranks in my college dorm years included the typical short-sheeting of beds and putting shaving cream on people's heads while they were sleeping. But the stories that Charles told went far beyond the typical college shenanigans. He and some of his friends once carried a classmate who slept very soundly out on his mattress to the middle of the campus courtyard and left him there, where he woke up the next morning.

During Charles's illness, a college friend of his sent an e-mail reminiscing about the crazy things they'd done. "Remember the time I tried to lock you overnight in the administration building," Charles's college friend wrote, "and I only left you with a candy bar and your Greek book? You called me from the front desk, still locked in the building. And when I went to check on you, you escaped past me out the front door and back to your room. I thought I had you that night, but you got out of it again."

This friend described how they had a running game of seeing who could pull the biggest practical joke on the other. "I'm afraid Charles won," he said, telling how Charles had put a live crab in his bed one night.

Charles had always had a good sense of humor, but not the silliness that this disease seemed to stimulate by removing some of his inhibitions. He'd never sung out loud spontaneously before. The disease brought out an almost sweet, childlike sense of fun. With his grim prognosis and constant physical deterioration, I cherished these small opportunities to laugh, and I think he did, too.

KEEPING CHARLES'S COMMITMENTS

Not wanting to give in to his disease, Charles remained committed to and active in his volunteer work in the business community.

Serving as business liaison on the Boston College steering committee of the Leadership for Change program created one venue for him to do this. He contributed not only his business savvy but also his passion and philosophy for people-centered leadership. When tensions arose, which can easily happen among academicians from such disparate departments as sociology and business management,

he skillfully intervened with just the right encouragement or admonition, allowing them to stay focused on their higher purpose of
creating a truly unique and powerful curriculum. Charles relished
the sense of community they all shared and the deep friendships
that developed.

He never stopped working with the New England chapter of the
ESOP Association, ensuring that the energy he had created for
employee ownership in New England did not fade, even as his own
abilities were slowly withering. He continued as best he could to
serve as its president, attend and lead meetings of the board of directors, and plan their conferences. But now he needed to rely on the
help of many others, who were fortunately all very willing to assist
this man they so greatly admired.

Because he now needed assistance with the daily activities of life, I
accompanied him to Las Vegas for the national association's semiannual board meeting, held at the MGM Grand Hotel on the weekend of a big Evander Holyfield boxing match. We struggled to
maneuver through the crowds to get to the board meeting. Once
there, he remained quiet for most of the meeting, waiting until the
end to express his opinion on the meeting's accomplishments. He
slurred his words inarticulately as he tried to praise the team for its
spirit of cooperation. After we arrived back at our hotel room, he
wilted with despair; he felt such frustration that he couldn't contribute to the discussions as he would have liked, and that he'd poorly verbalized his final thoughts.

However, months later at the annual conference, Michael, the
president of the ESOP Association, paid special tribute to Charles.
He praised Charles for his meaningful and encouraging words at the
last board of directors meeting; the same words that Charles felt had
been ineffective had actually resonated perfectly. Charles was certainly hard on himself. Others totally understood his struggles and
focused on the emotion behind the words, not on the manner in
which they were said.

Earlier in the year, Ilona and Janos of the Share-Participation
Foundation in Budapest, Hungary, invited Charles back for the fifth
time to consult with selected companies. Because of Charles's stiff-

ness and unstable balance, he wouldn't have traveled there if it hadn't been for Steve's willingness to personally help him. Steve, a close ESOP friend from Minneapolis, took responsibility in caring for Charles's needs on the trip. Steve handled all the baggage and even assisted Charles on his daily runs by holding his arm.

Even though Charles struggled to capture his thoughts in words and clearly articulate them when consulting with the Hungarian businesses, Janos assured us that Charles had nonetheless had an impact on the managers he'd addressed. And I know the time Charles had with Steve, Ilona, and Janos provided precious discussions, memories, and a lasting bond. My favorite picture from their trip showed Charles, who couldn't swim even before the onset of his symptoms, and Steve decked out in purple flowered bathing caps, sitting on the edge of one of the famous baths of Budapest, modern incarnations of people who have visited there over the centuries in hopes of healing. The two men hoped that the water's minerals would help Charles.

The day Charles returned from Hungary, March 17, 1997, he reached a huge milestone: one thousand days in a row of running, achieving his daily personal victory. He got congratulatory cards and plaques from Web Industries plants around the United States.

In all his commitments, whether to his personal goals or to promoting his deeply held convictions of caring leadership and employee ownership, Charles clearly found fulfillment in persevering, no matter what it took.

Caregiving Affirmation:
Find fulfillment in persevering with your loved one.

4

❦

1998: Then It Gets Worse

THE ADVENT OF AIDES

AIDES REQUIRED AT WORK

The managers at Web Industries accomplished what had been so difficult for me to do: They insisted that Charles have an aide at work.

I drove into Web one afternoon for our prescheduled appointment with the company leaders. We would meet with Donnie, the president; Al, the human resources manager; and Dan, the vice president for sales, who was also Charles's best friend and colleague at work. I assisted Charles as he walked apprehensively to sit at the big wooden table in Donnie's office. Donnie, smiling warmly, began. "We want you, Charles, to be able to work for as long as you can. And we know how important that is for you. However, Al and the administrative assistants can no longer provide the growing support you need and still accomplish their jobs. To continue working, we'll need you to have an aide. And to help financially, we can share the cost of the aide with you." Because Charles had no intention of retiring, he agreed.

I had already suspected that his growing decline would make an aide necessary at the office. Charles needed help not only to go to the cafeteria and restroom, but also to accomplish even the most mundane projects at work—dialing his phone, using his computer, and finding files. But I wouldn't have been able to convince him to get an aide without the intervention of the management team at Web. Whenever I had brought up the topic with Charles, he'd resisted. With Web's insistence, Charles would have to accept this latest sign of his growing disability.

I began the grueling task of searching for aides, calling one agency after another. Not only was there a severe shortage of aides in our area, but we would also require nonstandard expertise. The aide we needed would have to provide assistance with the basic skills of toileting, eating, and walking—and also serve as a quasi-secretary. The agencies argued that many aides weren't "suitable for a work environment." And our experience soon proved them right.

Finally, a contact at one of the half dozen agencies I called was willing to try and locate someone to meet our unique needs. The agency contact found a short-term solution while searching for a permanent one. Charles described Terry, his first female aide, as a "child." I never met her, but apparently the petite nursing student hardly looked old enough to be out of high school. Nevertheless, she performed her duties with expertise, carefully easing Charles into being comfortable with having a woman other than me take him to the restroom. Unfortunately, Terry stayed only two weeks because of the start of her full-time nursing program.

The agency replaced Terry with a red-haired, explosive permanent aide named Mary. A "tortured soul," as Charles would call her, Mary soon began to disturb the work environment—causing the administrative assistant to call me about bizarre events, including, believe it or not, Mary's carrying a gun. We didn't want the disruption of changing aides again, but this was just too much, so we asked that she be taken off our case.

Then our gem, Deedee, showed up. Tall and strong, with long blonde hair and bangs, large-framed glasses, and a pleasant attitude, Deedee fit in well in the office environment. She conscientiously took care of Charles—we couldn't have asked for a more dependable person. Deedee became comfortable with performing basic office tasks, even learning how to use a word-processing program. In just a short time, we realized that she could clearly handle both Charles's physical and professional needs.

But Deedee worked only Tuesdays through Fridays, meaning we still needed to find an aide for Mondays. The agency that had found Deedee searched, but came up with no one, so we started asking other agencies again—many whose representatives candidly said that filling our needs sounded impossible. Finally, one of them found Debbie.

While Debbie was pleasant, she showed up late nearly every day, shifting the responsibility of Charles's care to the office staff. Some days she just called in sick. Then she clearly crossed the line by trying to persuade Charles to give her money. We had to switch aides again.

This started the rotation of different aides covering Mondays over the next few months. Some would stay for one day, while others might last a month or two. Mondays continued to be a struggle, part of the accumulating difficulties in caring for Charles.

The Ammar Escapade

Even though we were already in our new house, Charles's needs were escalating at home, too. I now needed an aide for the after-work hours. I was exhausted from my routine of coming home after a full day at work, attending to Charles, making dinner, and then getting us both ready for bed. Tom, the EAP counselor, encouraged us to get help, and suggested we try hiring our own aide.

My innate caution had led me to suspect that not going through an agency had risks. But I didn't listen to that caution, because hiring on our own would cost about half as much as going through agencies. At the time, most organizations charged seventeen dollars an hour—but we could probably hire on our own for nine to ten dollars an hour. We also thought that we could save some money if we offered the evening aide the opportunity to move into one of our empty upstairs bedrooms. We could deduct the value of rent and utilities from the hourly payment for the services. That would also provide the advantage of having someone in the house if we had an emergency with Charles during the night.

We posted a job description at various colleges. With some assistance from the counselor, we also prepared an ad for the local newspapers and *The Boston Globe*.

LIVE-IN HEALTH AIDE
Framingham. Young handicapped corp. exec. with progressive
neurological disorder seeks assistance w/home care needs such
as toileting, showering, cooking, laundry. Home health aide
or equivalent preferred. Nonsmkr. 20+ hrs/wk, primarily
early evening and possibly wkd hours. Compet. sal. & 2 rms
w/lg bath. Call . . .

At the same time, Gerard had announced that he would be starting a full-time job and soon would be unable to continue his work
with us. Gerard, once acting as a driver only, had recently been getting Charles ready for work in the mornings. My sister Barb had suggested this idea when we moved into the apartment. Gerard was a
former student nurse, so I knew he would have the ability. I was
thrilled, and terribly relieved, when he agreed. Now I hoped that the
new evening aide we found would also be able to take on the morning duties when Gerard left. I wanted to avoid the arduous additional work of interviewing and hiring another aide just for the morning.

My mom had been visiting when our ad appeared in the paper.
Because she was home during the day, she took the initial phone
calls from interested candidates. I prepared questions for her to ask
on the phone before inviting the candidate in for an interview:

- Why are you interested in the job?
- What experience do you have?
- What training, certification, or education have you had?
- Do you have any experience dealing with someone who has
  a serious illness?

If a candidate passed this first screen, Mom asked the person to
come for an interview and bring a résumé (or work history), references, and certification card.

One night, she told me that a candidate named Ammar had
proactively said, "When do you want me to start?" He wanted the
job. When I later interviewed him, his wife Farah came with him.
Ammar was a huge man from Nigeria. He was a bit gruff, but nice
enough. Farah, on the other hand, was sweet and polite. Before

starting, though, Ammar asked, "How's Charles?" which I considered thoughtful.

During this interview, as in all the other interviews I conducted, I made requests such as these:

- Describe how you safely showered a patient who had stability problems.
- Show me the techniques you use to assist a patient in walking, using me as an example.
- Show me examples of range-of-motion exercises you have done for another client.
- Give me an example of how you deal with stress.

Then I inquired about certifications and references.

After the interview, Ammar summarized why I should hire him. "I'm dependable, hardworking, and truthful. Farah and I go to church each Sunday, to the Baptist church." Both Ammar and Farah claimed they had home health aide certification. Though I would be hiring Ammar, Farah was willing to help when she could. I would almost be getting two aides for the price of one.

My sister Carolyn, in Florida, checked three references for each of our top candidates. When she called me with her summary, she said, "Hire Darry." Darry had been my top choice from the interviews, and Carolyn had received glowing reports from his references. They thought highly of Darry and couldn't say enough good things about him. But he had a full-time job, so he wouldn't be able to take over for Gerard in the mornings. Though Ammar's references didn't give glowing recommendations, no one said anything that caused us concern. One commented that he was professional. Another mentioned that he performed satisfactorily. And because he was unemployed, he could take over the morning routine once Gerard left.

I hired Ammar.

It didn't take long for things to go wrong. Every morning before work, I gave Charles a twenty-dollar bill to pay for his breakfast and lunch. He would come home with the change each evening. The first night that Ammar cared for Charles, the change was missing. I said to Ammar, "Charles usually brings home change in his pocket. Did you find it when you undressed him?" "No," he replied quite emphatically, feigning to look for the change in Charles's pocket, to no avail.

The next night when I came home from work, Ammar had left Charles's change on our bedroom bureau. It was not only the change from that day but also from the day before! He didn't say anything. In fact, I don't think he even realized that I had recognized his lie. I would have fired Ammar right then, but because of Charles's caring nature and reluctance to give up on him, I allowed Ammar to stay. Even though confrontation is very difficult for me, I gathered my courage and spoke with him about the importance of trust in our relationship.

As the week progressed, my cleaning woman and my decorator, both of whom had work to do in the house during the day, had called me. In the course of the conversation, they expressed that Ammar had frightened them, ordering them around and making them feel uncomfortable.

The last straw came when early one morning, Ammar actually came into our bedroom while we were still sleeping. I heard him. When I asked what he was doing, he jerked around and quickly picked up a laundry basket in our closet and said that he was doing the wash. Obviously it was not appropriate to enter our bedroom with both of us still in bed. And my suspicions of other motives escalated when I saw my purse sitting close to the laundry baskets.

I finally talked Charles into letting him go, so later that morning, Charles and I took him to breakfast at a café. I didn't want to fire him while we were at home. That felt too vulnerable. Doing it around other people seemed safer. While we were conversing at breakfast, I learned a lot about Nigeria from Ammar. He was very open about the corruption there and also about his family's ties to the government. He also mentioned that he had dual citizenship. While Farah lived full-time in America, he spent much of the year in Nigeria.

As we finished breakfast, in a nervous voice that I couldn't control, I fired Ammar and told him that we wanted him to move out immediately. He argued and tried to talk us into keeping him on— at least until the next day. I get scared even now thinking about what he would have tried to accomplish overnight at our house. Thankfully, Ammar did move out that day.

Our ordeal was over—or so we thought. Shortly after Ammar and Farah had left, we received our phone bill: a whopping $788.06 in calls to Nigeria! And they took place over only six days. Obviously, Ammar had had no intention of staying with us for the long term.

I got some of our money back by calling Farah at work. She and I agreed that she would send us fifty dollars each week. I got only one hundred dollars from her, but I didn't have the strength to push any further.

I still have fears about my financial accounts. Ammar had access to all of my personal folders during the day. My financial planner advised me long ago to get locked cabinets, but that was one more task to do—and frankly, I had plenty to do just taking care of Charles. Shortly after Ammar left, though, I made the time to buy locked file cabinets and moved all of my financial records into them.

We'd taken all the right steps in the hiring process—conducting interviews, confirming home health aide certification, and checking references—but still had a terrifying, draining experience.

The evening that I fired Ammar, I called Darry to see if he was still available and wanted the job—and he did. We hired him for the evening shift and allowed him to move into our upstairs living space. Darry turned out to be extremely loyal, reliable, caring, and patient, and he had a great sense of humor. He drove Charles home from work each night, then helped with the evening tasks.

When Gerard stopped working in the mornings, an agency found Carlos—a stocky, compassionate aide from Brazil. He prepared Charles for his day and also drove him to work each morning.

Caregiving Affirmation:
Anticipate difficulty in finding dependable home health aides.

CHARLES WRITES HIS BOOK

One day back in 1996, we had just finished our run. As I held Charles's arm tightly to assist him up the stairs of our Newton house, I initiated one of our significant conversations. Though it was always hard for me to bring up anything that dealt with the short amount of time he had left in life, it just felt right that day. I asked, "With this disease, Charles, is there anything you wish you could have done, but haven't yet?"

Without hesitation, Charles said, "Yes. I have a book that I want to write." Decisively, he described it as being about leadership. "I thought of the idea when I was preparing my presentation as a guest speaker for Ginny's management class at the University of Pennsylvania. As I wove some of my old speeches together into this lecture, I discovered some paradoxes in my leadership philosophy. I tried them out on the students there, and they really worked."

"That sounds like an interesting and unique way to approach leadership," I said. "Have you thought of a title for the book?"

"My working title is *Paradoxes of Leadership*," he said resolutely.

Making the book happen became our next struggle. Charles continued to work long hours at Web Industries, while also putting in volunteer hours with the employee ownership community. He served as president of the New England ESOP Association, as a member of the board of directors of the national ESOP Association, and as facilitator for the national group's strategic planning committee. And he still traveled internationally to talk about employee ownership and leadership. With his increasing disability, all of these activities took more effort than before. When would he find time to write his book?

Later that year, we visited Charles's younger brother Ken in Arkansas. Ken seemed to find it easy to raise the difficult issues that I often struggled to bring up with Charles. We enjoyed the best conversations sitting in Ken's small, country-style living room. "The journey is now," Ken repeated frequently, encouraging Charles to live each day to the fullest and to not procrastinate in fulfilling his dreams. "What do you want to do now, before the disease progresses?" Ken asked directly. Feeling put on the spot by Ken's persistence,

Charles finally shared the idea for his book. That was all Ken needed to hear. From that point on, Ken asked Charles, in his almost weekly calls, "How's the book coming? Have you started it yet?" Ken didn't stop pestering even though it took months for Charles to begin.

I felt guilty that I didn't take the time to sit with Charles at the computer to help him start writing, but I was too overwhelmed with my job and the increasing responsibility of caring for him. All I could do was try to figure out a way to get Charles started. It wasn't that Charles didn't want to begin writing the book; it was just that we still tended to live our lives as if he didn't have a disease, which made it easy to procrastinate.

Finally, though, in late 1997, Charles committed to start writing. This was at a time when he often felt unable to effectively complete tasks at work, so he would use some of his time at the office to type his thoughts. Unfortunately, this was also when he started to lose the ability for his eyes to follow lines of text on the computer screen and to pick out the correct letters on the keyboard.

Later, we decided to ask Deedee to help. Charles could dictate his thoughts, and Deedee could type them into the computer. She found this awkward at first because she was just beginning to learn how to use word-processing software, and was even less knowledgeable about business and leadership. On my morning runs with Charles, I tried to assist by asking him to tell me about a story from his work experience that illustrated one of the paradoxes. When we would get home from a run, I would jot the story down for Charles to take to work.

Deedee began to capture Charles's words in a document, but she lacked the expertise to organize the random ideas into a coherent outline. We were happy when Loren volunteered to help.

While Deedee didn't have the depth of business knowledge necessary to understand the themes Charles tried to convey, Loren did. Charles also seemed more comfortable working with Loren for this project because Loren worked for him as the part-time administrator of the New England chapter of the ESOP Association. For over eight months, Loren selflessly devoted one day each weekend to the project. Because he didn't own a car, he took a bus, subway, and train to Framingham, where I picked him up at the station. Loren keyed in

Charles's new thoughts, reworked pieces Deedee had typed, and kept the process moving forward. We wouldn't have been able to complete the book without Loren's dedicated assistance.

As time progressed, though, Charles began to lose the ability to recall stories. We knew he had many more leadership vignettes in his head, but the disease prevented him from retrieving them. In addition, Charles was losing the ability to articulate his thoughts well enough to be understood. Even Deedee, who was able to interpret Charles's garbled speech longer than anyone else, struggled to decipher what he was saying.

Eventually, Loren could only take the passages that he or Deedee had already typed and elaborate on them. Charles, with a simple yes or no, would indicate his approval or disapproval for what Loren had written. Eventually, we all had to admit that what we had was all we were going to get, and that it would have to be enough.

Loren and I solicited the help of other volunteers to get Charles's book printed. Corey, the director of the National Center for Employee Ownership, organized the raw sections into the appropriate chapters. He also spent many hours editing the book, doing the layout, and coordinating the other necessary steps for publication, such as getting the ISBN and registering the copyright. To cover the printing expenses, Loren and Corey solicited commitments from employee-owned companies to buy multiple copies of the book.

Clay, another friend, volunteered to design the cover. Clay worked for Delta Airlines at the time as a graphic artist. He produced a truly professional and creative cover, depicting the concept of paradoxes with a rock and a feather.

Writing and publishing *Paradoxes of Leadership* fulfilled an important goal for Charles. It also gave him a sense of value, because he could now do so little. Later in the disease when he couldn't talk or communicate, I enjoyed seeing his eyes open wide with attention every time I read him an e-mail from someone touched by the book. Charles passionately wanted to fulfill his mission to make a difference in the world; his book allowed him to accomplish this goal, even when his body was starting to fail him.

Paradoxes of Leadership preserved his philosophy of valuing each individual in the workplace by listening and caring. He started his book with the words from the old 1960s song "Five O'Clock World,"recorded by the Vogues: "It's a five o'clock world when the whistle blows/No one owns a piece of my time." Charles was disturbed about this though. As he would say, "Too many people are selling their lives away for a paycheck and don't find meaning in their jobs." His book tried to encourage managers to adopt leadership principles that value the individual.

And Charles lived these paradoxes. The first paradox he wrote about—*We have more influence when we listen than when we tell*—exemplifies his most powerful interpersonal skill. When he first started to hone this paradox, I remember his brown eyes looking intently into mine as he asked, "Janet, how do you feel when someone *tells* you what to do?" Then he probed further: "What does a teenager instinctively do when a parent tells him what to do? He'll do the opposite. Nobody likes someone telling them what to do." To counterbalance the telling, Charles promoted the concept of deep listening. He could masterfully ask questions that allowed others to learn for themselves.

Another paradox described Charles's character: *We correct better through grace than through confrontation.* "Nobody sets out to be a jerk," he'd explain. "If someone does something wrong, assume the best." He felt that people would rise and fall to our expectations of them. And Charles always seemed to live by the principle of grace at home and at work.

When he saw the first printed copy of *Paradoxes of Leadership* in late 1998, Charles couldn't physically express his excitement—by that point, the disease prevented his emotions from showing on his face. Although I held the cover up right in front of his eyes, I'm not certain he could see it in total. But he listened intently when I read the touching preface written by his friend Steve, CEO of an employee-owned company, which concluded: "If *Paradoxes of Leadership* helps even one reader to understand, accept, and improve leadership effectiveness, it will be a leadership lesson of the highest order, given from the perspective of a full life and from the heart of Charles's final paradox: *A full life is achieved not by grasping, but by giving.* Charles has given us a gift for the new millennium, and beyond. . . ."

I doubt Charles would have ever made the time to write a book if this neurological disease hadn't struck. What would have slowed his pre-disease life schedule enough to give him the time and impetus to write? His disease gave him the gift of his book.

Caregiving Affirmation:
Don't be shy about asking others for assistance.
Their willingness to help may astound you.

OUR NEW DAILY ROUTINE

Rolling onto the floor from my makeshift bed—an old comforter folded up for a mattress—I started our day.

I'd begun sleeping on the floor next to our bed when Charles's fidgeting and insomnia kept me awake most of the night. On one of my first attempts to move onto the floor, Charles yelled, "You don't want to sleep with me anymore!" He didn't understand. To him, the change meant that I was rejecting him. But that wasn't true at all. I longed for the close times we'd had each night, falling asleep with our bodies snuggled tightly together. By this point in Charles's disease, I couldn't sleep while he struggled to keep still during the night. As time went on, I slipped out of bed and onto the floor after Charles seemed to be asleep. I had hoped he wouldn't notice, even though I really knew that he did. I didn't want to hurt his feelings, but I needed sleep. The hard floor allowed more restful sleep than the bed, which kept shifting all night with Charles's syncopated movements.

Eventually, at my mom's suggestion, I replaced the comforter with cushions from our big fold-out couch upstairs, and later, with an inflatable mattress donated by my friend, Jean.

But moving permanently to the floor didn't give me the full night's sleep that I needed. Charles, unable to help himself in any way, woke me up like clockwork every hour to turn him over or attend to him in some other way. I understand that we sleep in nine-

ty-minute cycles, which allows our bodies to get into the deep sleep
we need for rejuvenation. Waking up before getting thoroughly into
each cycle of deep sleep can have devastating effects—both emotional and physical—and can feel like torture. And to make it worse, I
had found it hard, with stressful thoughts swimming through my
head each night, to go back to sleep after Charles woke me up. I
started taking one or two Tylenol PM pills so that I could at least fall
back asleep once I'd been awakened.

My hourly wake-up calls lasted nearly the entire year. I don't
know how I functioned during the day at work. My sympathetic
staff contributed more than required to fill the gap created by my
difficulties. And they always proactively offered to help, keeping our
busy department's projects moving ahead on time. Though I came
home exhausted each night, I tried to remain cheerful while under-
taking my evening tasks. My getting through that grueling period
must have been a testament to my defense mechanisms. All of us
have these inner defenses in the midst of trauma. We don't seem to
break down until after the crisis is over. Nonetheless, I'm sure I
walked around like a zombie each day.

"Why don't you move into a different room?" friends would ask.
I just wasn't ready for that yet. If I left the room, I would feel as if I
really were abandoning Charles. And besides, he still would have
awakened every hour and called out for me to attend to him. I could
do that more easily by sleeping on the floor next to him instead of
down the hall in another room.

Once awake and dressed for our run, I would load Charles into the
car and we'd drive down the street to the nearby apartment complex.
We'd run, my arm in his, back and forth inside the covered concrete
and brick parking lot sheltered from the rain, wind, and snow. We
didn't practice speech exercises as much anymore. Instead, we would
strategize about his book—what story he could write about that day—
or how else he could contribute at work.

After we returned, Charles would slur the words *Eye Opener,*
reminding me to turn on his favorite early morning news show after
I had put him on the toilet. He struggled with his bowel movements,
sitting on the toilet for thirty to sixty minutes. I felt that that

amount of time was excessive and the reason for his painful hemor-
rhoids, but I couldn't talk him into getting up sooner. It was enough
time, though, for me to quickly shower before Gerard arrived.

Gerard would take full charge of getting Charles ready for work,
starting with getting him off the toilet. Charles's muscle stiffness
kept him standing very erect while Gerard wiped his buttocks,
another essential ability that Charles had recently lost. We had
heard about this humiliating limitation when watching the tape of
Morrie Schwartz's interview with Ted Koppel on *Nightline*. (Morrie
is the main character of the book *Tuesdays with Morrie*.) Morrie
called it the "ass wiping" test, a milestone in the neurological losses
he would experience with amyotrophic lateral sclerosis (Lou
Gehrig's) disease. Charles had already reached this milestone in his
disease's progression.

Gerard even gave Charles a new hairstyle. He combed it straight
back, instead of the right part and side sweep across his forehead that
Charles had been doing for years. I didn't like the new look at first,
but I eventually realized that it made Charles look distinguished and
classy, befitting his personality.

Charles ate his breakfast—dry muesli or low-fat granola cereal
out of a red plastic cup—in the car on the way to work. He could
still hold the cup himself but was beginning to lose some of the
coordination needed to keep the dry cereal from spilling onto the
seat and floor of the car.

With Deedee, the aide at work, attending to him all day, he had
official help getting around—to and from the lunchroom, conference room, and restroom. It didn't take long for Deedee and the
other aides to know to order Charles the turkey roll-up sandwich
with cranberry sauce and a fruit cup for lunch. The cafeteria owner,
who knew Charles personally, began to fix "the usual" as soon as
she saw him walk in. He'd been ordering this same lunch from the
time he couldn't read the menu over a year ago. And now, Deedee
would get Charles a straw for his diet iced tea each day, which kept
spills to a minimum.

I packed Charles's daytime pills in a plastic pillbox at the beginning of each week so that the aide could assist Charles in taking

them. To reduce confusion, I provided an up-to-date list of medications, describing the color and size of each pill, and when Charles should take it.

During the workday, though, Charles faced increasing frustrations. His body grew increasingly stiff and inflexible in his office chair. And adding to the irritation, his tightened muscles kept his body's temperature control out of whack. "My feet are hot," Charles would say for the hundredth time. It wasn't just in his mind; even in the dead of winter, we would dress him with a golf shirt, though everyone else had on warm wool sweaters. We bought a small portable fan to blow on him during work to keep him from burning up. Even so, I found his shirt often drenched with sweat when he got home.

But those amounted to only the physical discomforts Charles faced while at work. Because of Charles's incontinence, accidents still happened, even though Deedee automatically took him to the restroom every two to three hours and changed his pads. I packed a change of underwear and pants that we kept at work in a plastic bag for those unfortunate and embarrassing times.

Charles's vision and movement problems made it impossible for him to keep up with his job as he should, and he knew it. I'd work with him at home to organize his main projects. But I knew that once he was at work, he couldn't really accomplish any of the tasks required to move these projects along effectively. He even struggled with his mentoring calls to the plant managers—the job activity he'd always found the most meaningful. Charles's brain seemed to block the retrieval of the right words to say, reducing the effectiveness of his counseling. And people began to find it difficult to understand his garbled speech, except for his final phrase, "How can I support you?" As the year progressed, Charles revealed his fear to me: "I think they are going to force me to retire."

One way that Charles found meaning in his work came from sending "daily thoughts" via e-mail to people he wanted to affect. Tom, the employee assistance counselor Charles and I were seeing, wisely suggested that doing this could help counteract Charles's depression at his dwindling ability to contribute to work and life. To facilitate this, Deedee spent an hour or two each day reading leadership books, such as *Leadership Is an Art* and *Emotional Intelligence: Why It Can Matter More Than IQ*, out loud to him. When Charles liked a particular passage, he'd mumble to her, "Thought for the day," and she'd underline it for inclusion in a future e-mail message.

Deedee helped Charles pass the time of day by playing books on tape. By that point, Charles was legally blind because of his limited field of vision. When asked what he could see, he'd say, "I can see everything." But the neuro-ophthalmologist's tests showed he had lost much of his peripheral vision. This diagnosis made him eligible for free resources. The National Library of Congress provided a special tape player and catalog of books on tape from which we made selections. To add some recreation to the day, Deedee took Charles for a walk in the morning and afternoon, which later in the year evolved to pushing Charles in a wheelchair.

Once home at night, we'd eat a frozen dinner and then head out for our daily frozen yogurt. Leaving Charles in the car, I would run in to get his favorite—a waffle cone with chocolate frozen yogurt on the bottom, M&Ms in the middle, and white chocolate mousse on top. Holding both of our cones, I would awkwardly lay out napkins, covering Charles from neck to knees. During our ride home, much of the yogurt dripped down his face onto his chest and lap. Acknowledging his yogurt-covered face when we arrived home always gave us a chuckle. Enjoying this frozen treat together gave us the most pleasure of the entire day.

Caregiving Affirmation:
Remember to enjoy the little things in life.

PHYSICAL CHALLENGES TEST EMOTIONAL STRENGTH

FIGHTING POISON WITH POISON

Before Botox gained popularity for cosmetic purposes, it showed promise in people like Charles who have conditions that cause muscles to contract beyond what is normal. At the PSP symposium, we had learned that some patients who had difficulty keeping their eyelids open found success with Botox shots. "Even though you are injecting poison into the body, it is not harmful in the doses we recommend," the neuro-ophthalmologist explained. "The botulism shots cause the muscles to relax by semiparalyzing them. But you do need to repeat the treatment every few weeks, as the effect does not last permanently."

The tightness in Charles's right calf muscle began to affect his ability to jog, prohibiting his heel from hitting the ground. We convinced him that walking could count for his daily personal victory. But even with just walking, he now always needed someone to hold his arm as the calf tightness threw his balance off so much that it became difficult to keep him stable. We wanted to do anything possible to help him maintain his mobility and his promise to himself to complete his daily personal victory. So I asked Dr. Ravin, "Do you think we could try Botox shots in Charles's calf muscles? Would that release them enough to allow him to walk more easily?"

"Let's give it a try," she responded, and then provided us with a referral.

Initially, it appeared that the shots helped. The doctor treated not only Charles's right calf but also his left one, as well as his arms, which had started to contract at the elbows. Charles never complained about the pain of the shots, and the nurse always commented on Charles's sweet nature. But after a few months, not even Botox could stop the brain's command to tighten the muscles.

OUT OF CONTROL WITH A WALKER

With my growing concern for Charles's safety, we needed to try something else.

The physical therapist who spoke at the PSP symposium suggested weighted walkers. These have three wheels, with the majority of their weight in the front of the device. The handlebars have brake levers similar to those on a ten-speed bike. Surely this should work for Charles, we thought. A number of the people with PSP at the symposium seemed to be using it effectively. And we had found that shopping carts in grocery stores worked well for him.

The medical supply store delivered a shiny green walker with a black seat that could fold down if Charles needed to stop and rest. With our long driveway in front of us, I placed Charles behind the walker and put his hands on the handlebars. I continued to hold his arm as I said, "Okay, Charles, you can start walking."

Once he began, the walker started to go faster than his feet could keep up. His upper body leaned forward, his feet trailing. "Can you use the brake to stop it?" I asked. Without responding, he continued out of control. I grabbed the walker with my free hand and stopped everything, until I could get Charles back in position to try again. Every time we tried, the walker sped faster than his feet. He didn't have the coordination to keep the walker close to him and use it as support for his walking. By the time we made it to the end of the driveway, he was yelling, "I can't do this!"

Now I had run out of options to keep him mobile.

Defiance in the Face of Unquestionable Disability

Getting Charles from place to place by walking became painstakingly slow. Step by step, we'd nearly waddle to our destination. Thankfully, I now had a HANDICAPPED placard that allowed me to park in those close-to-the-building handicapped spaces. But even at that, it took us a long time to get anywhere. And this limited where we could go. Charles's world was shrinking.

I asked him if he'd consider a wheelchair. "It will give you much more mobility," I said. "Just think—we could go to the mall and stroll past the shops. And we could even go to a museum." I can't remember if he really agreed, but I at least interpreted some signs of approval. So when the medical supply store picked up the walker, I had them deliver a wheelchair. Charles showed a bit of frustration while the deliveryman demonstrated how the attachments worked and how the soft extra seat cushion would mold to Charles's shape, giving him maximum comfort.

The second the man left, Charles screamed in defiance, "I'm not handicapped! I don't need this!" Just like when I had initiated the use of the incontinence pads, I had become the bad guy, introducing something that further highlighted his disability.

"But Charles, the wheelchair will allow us to take you to more places. It will give you more freedom." This line of reasoning didn't work right away. Charles continued his frustrated rebellion for a while. But eventually, the wheelchair won out when Charles admitted that his need for it was greater than his distaste at using such a clear symbol of his disability. With the ease of pushing him wherever we wanted to go, we could enjoy a new sense of independence.

Caregiving Affirmation:
A new world of freedom will open up once your loved one agrees to use a wheelchair.

CONTINUED SAFETY CONCERNS

Being in a wheelchair and having aides for support didn't eliminate Charles's problem with falls. We all continued to be surprised by his instability.

With Charles holding onto the handicap rail in the bathroom one morning, an aide turned away. Before the aide knew it, Charles fell directly on his head, getting a cut large enough to require stitches. Another time, Charles fell from his shower chair when an aide thought he was stable, once again cutting his head.

Charles's instability showed up even in bed. I worried that he might shift enough to fall out, so I put pillows on the nightstand next to the bed to keep him from cutting himself on its corners if he did fall. The one time he fell out of bed, the pillow served the purpose I intended, but he hit his head on the bottom molding, cutting a gash that required yet another trip to the emergency room for stitches. The nurse at one of the agencies finally recommended an obvious solution—getting a full body pillow to put between Charles and the edge of the bed. That worked.

The other hazard we continually faced was Charles's stiff body slipping out of his wheelchair. The aides and I always placed him with his feet snugly in the footrests. But as we would push him through the house, neighborhood, or mall, his legs would eventually straighten, scooting off the footrests. That shifted his center of gravity, causing him to slide off the wheelchair toward the ground. One time, while I was at home alone with him, he slipped completely out of the wheelchair just before I got him into the bedroom. As hard as I tried, I could not get him back into the wheelchair. In desperation,

I finally had to call my neighbor for assistance. And even for two people, it was a struggle to place Charles back in the wheelchair. The agency recommended using a cloth seat belt. That helped, but it still wasn't foolproof. We eventually also needed to strap his ankles to the footrest with cloth belts.

The aides and I finally learned how to take care of Charles's safety needs. I only wish we could have done more to improve his comfort.

I can't imagine how awful it must have been for him to deal with his stiffness.

MANAGING (OR MISMANAGING) URINARY INCONTINENCE

I can't stand it anymore! I screamed mentally. The urine had gone everywhere.

I used a plastic Solo cup instead of a urinal when I took Charles to the bathroom, as it worked as well as a urinal and took up less space. I had put the filled cup of on the edge of the sink while I pulled up Charles's pants, zipped them, and then set him back in his wheelchair. But as I turned to pick up the cup and pour the urine into the toilet, I accidentally knocked it off the sink, sending the urine like a waterfall throughout this small handicapped restroom stall at the movie theater. As it hit the floor, it splashed up onto my pants and Charles's. On my hands and knees, I used paper towel after paper towel to wipe up the foul stuff.

Another time, we had just arrived at our car in the parking garage in downtown Boston. "I have to pee," Charles said. Once he admitted this, I needed to act quickly. I didn't have much time. I opened the car door to hide him from view, stood him up, and prepared to have him urinate into a plastic cup. But he started before I could get the cup in place. The urine went everywhere. And I'm embarrassed to say that without any paper towels to clean it up, I put Charles back in the car and we just drove off.

I had now dealt with one too many incidents with urine.

Over the previous couple of years, urinary incontinence had constantly challenged Charles's independence and strong will. He graduated from the simple men's pads to full Depends briefs. He wouldn't hear of making that change when I first brought it up. But one night he said to me, "Deedee said we should try the green pads that fit like underwear," not realizing those were the ones I had been trying to persuade him to try. I suppose it's sometimes easier to hear things from someone you're not married to; Deedee was Charles's favorite aide.

But even with the new briefs, there were still frequent accidents. The briefs are marketed to the elderly; I suppose that senior men don't have the same volume of urine as a man in his forties. The medical supply store recommended that we add Dignity brand pads to our regimen. They were like triple-size sanitary napkins. We put two of them in the front of the briefs to help absorb the urine.

Around the house, in the car, and at work, I always had Charles sit on an underpad so that the furniture, car seat, and his wheelchair wouldn't get soiled. "What are you doing? I don't need that," he'd say in embarrassment if he saw me put the underpad down while someone else was around. I continued, though, as I couldn't fathom the additional cleanup effort that would have been required without them. When he had an accident, I'd again be dealing with wet pants, underclothes, and underpad. And even when we made it to the bathroom, Charles couldn't control the direction of urine flow into the toilet, which meant I had to do daily cleanups on my hands and knees.

Because of our continued busy lifestyle—going to work, restaurants, movies, and other events—I was always prepared. I bought a black wheelchair backpack, had it embroidered with Charles's name, and packed it full of supplies—a plastic cup, extra Depends pads, Gold Bond medicated powder, clean underpad, plastic bag for dirty items, and Handi Wipes and latex gloves for cleanup.

Whether in the airport or at my office, I wheeled Charles into the women's restroom. The women there tried to ignore the man who had just entered, but I didn't have much choice. Rarely could I find a family or handicapped single restroom. At least I knew that Charles probably couldn't see much because of his lack of peripheral vision. And it wasn't an option for me to take him into the men's restroom.

Our process was the same every time. I rolled Charles into the handicapped stall, facing the toilet. I took the plastic cup out of the pack and placed it at my feet. Then I put his left hand on the handicapped railing. Grabbing under his arms, I lifted him to a stand. Continuing with my arms around him so that he could lean on my left shoulder, I unzipped his pants and pulled them down. Then I reached for the cup, put it in place, and hoped for success.

Another constant struggle was that Charles would deny needing to go to the restroom if I asked. He even got mad at me when I tried to persuade him that we had an opportunity that we should take advantage of. Then when he finally did need to go, it was often too late. Once again, our different personalities put us at odds: I'm the organized one, always thinking ahead; Charles always preferred to wing it.

But none of that came close to the emotional trauma Charles and I experienced at bedtime with the condom catheter. The Depends briefs with the Dignity pads would not last through the night, so we needed another solution. We'd heard about condom catheters, so we decided to try one.

The medical supply store first asked what size condom we needed. I had no idea. If I got one too small, it would probably squeeze and hurt Charles. Too big, and it wouldn't stay on. So I tried medium. The sales representative made them sound easy to use. Simply open the package, roll one on, and then hook it to the tube that is attached to the catheter bag. I decided I'd give it a try.

Charles screamed in pain as I rolled one on. "It hurts!"

"Let's see how it feels once we have it on," I replied. I honestly didn't think he needed a large size. The medium should fit fine, I thought.

Once I had it on and hooked up to the catheter bag, I needed to find a place to hang the bag. The tube should be extended so the urine could flow unimpeded, using gravity. In a hospital, there would have been a number of bars to hang it on. But Charles was still sleeping in our own bed. I tried a variety of options, eventually pinning it to the mattress sheet.

We were all set. Charles continued to complain, but I convinced him to give it a try overnight. We did make it through the first night, but when I took off the condom the next morning, numerous pubic hairs rolled down within it. "Owwww!" Charles exclaimed. I had no doubt his pain was real.

I found this problem difficult to solve. Shaving seemed senseless, as it would need to be done regularly to keep the newly grown stubble from irritating him. I'm not sure how I got the idea, but I tore a bunch of his old T-shirts into strips. I wrapped one around the bottom of the condom to keep the hairs out of the way. That mostly worked. But every now and then, a hair would get caught and pinch Charles with pain.

It wasn't long before a condom came completely off one night, soaking the sheets. We struggled to get the catheter bag in a position that would allow a smooth flow. The entire process required a delicate balance that I never could be certain had been reached until the next morning, which was too late.

"Why do you make me wear these?" Charles complained every night when we prepared to put one on. "I can't have you wetting the sheets night after night. I don't know what else to do," I said, desperate. Charles hated this process, and I hated it, too. But no matter how loudly he yelled or how hard he protested, I still put it on, believing I had no other choice.

My friend Mickey, working on his degree in medicine, told me that incontinence is one of the major reasons caregivers choose to put someone in a nursing home. I can understand why—I was totally exasperated with this issue. But I was still determined to keep Charles home and manage this seemingly unmanageable problem as best I could.

Caregiving Affirmation:
Handling the most basic caregiving needs can be draining,
so seek the advice of experts to lighten your load.

EXERTING HIS STRONG WILL

STUBBORNNESS

For some reason, Charles became more stubborn as the disease progressed. He certainly had always had a bit of a stubborn streak, which I think he got from his mother. But it usually came out only when I was trying to make him do something he didn't want to do. Now he adamantly insisted on certain things, and often they didn't even make sense to me—which is what made them hard to deal with emotionally.

For example, when we were interviewing a potential aide named Junior, Charles insisted on going upstairs to see the second floor of our new Framingham home. He was still walking at the time, but I could no longer handle him alone going upstairs. Junior must have weighed only one hundred twenty pounds soaking wet. I feared that he, too, wouldn't be strong enough to assist. And what was the point? I was pretty sure that Charles couldn't even see well enough once he made it upstairs. Also, climbing stairs with Charles wouldn't be one of Junior's duties if we hired him. Our main goal at the moment was to interview Junior to see if he would be a good fit as an aide—caring and capable of providing basic needs, such as assistance in walking and showering.

"This would be a serious safety risk," I argued. "The steps are slippery and narrow. It would be too hard to get you upstairs." Nonetheless, Charles insisted, nearly yelling at me, "I want to go upstairs and look around." So Junior and I squeezed on either side of Charles and wiggled our way to the top of the stairs. Once up, we easily toured Charles around the bedrooms and bathroom. But coming down was much scarier. If Charles had gotten off balance, I'm not sure that Junior and I would have been able to prevent a fall. Somehow we made it. I wasn't surprised that Junior never returned our calls after that experience.

Upon reflection, I wonder if Charles was just being stubborn at the time or if he felt this was a good test of Junior's ability to handle him physically. Or maybe he realized that his only opportunity to see the rest of the house would be during an interview with a potential new aide. Or maybe an effect of his disease was fixation on what would normally be passing fancies. At the time, though, all I heard was a stubborn, angry man.

Then there was the dumbbell incident. Though it wasn't a real problem and certainly wasn't as embarrassing as the Junior incident, it was still puzzling and frustrating. Charles demanded that we get hand weights so that he could do strength exercises. This would have made a lot of sense if he was able to move his arms at will, but he couldn't. I tried to talk him out of getting them—arguing that he wouldn't be able to use them—but he continued to insist. I finally pushed him into Sears in his wheelchair and bought one-pound iron dumbbells.

I wondered if his motivation was concern about me. Maybe he thought that if we had the weights, I would use them. I had recently been having difficulty transferring him on my own. And I would tell him that I just wasn't strong enough to meet his needs. I think he was scared about what it would mean if I couldn't move him, and therefore, couldn't care for him.

At the time, both of these incidents totally aggravated and frustrated me. I could see no rational explanation for his stubbornness and insistence. But in reflecting on it now as I write, I realize that if Charles did have ulterior motives for his requests, he just didn't, or couldn't, let me know what they were.

OBSESSIONS

What could be happening in his brain to cause so many obsessions? I wondered. It seemed lately that whenever Charles latched onto something, he couldn't get enough of it.

Earlier in the disease, he'd obsessed about time, and the fear of being late. Now he had developed a Beatles mania. He had always liked the Beatles, but he'd rarely gone out of his way to listen to their music. Now, however, he insisted on hearing the one cassette tape of the Beatles greatest hits music that we owned over and over. When I was around, I'd sing along with "She Loves You," "Hey Jude," and "I Want to Hold Your Hand." Other times when I'd had enough, he'd listen to them through earphones. This wasn't just a passing fancy for Charles—he was addicted. "Beatles," Charles would slur to let me know he wanted his fix. I bought more of their CDs, including *A Hard Day's Night, Magical Mystery Tour,* and *Sgt. Pepper's Lonely Hearts Club Band.* One weekend, I rented the *Beatles Anthology* on video, and finally, I bought a set to help satisfy his desire.

Charles also became obsessed with a song by Jewel, "Foolish Games." He made me buy the CD, and we played it a couple of times each night. We'd listen as Jewel sang "These foolish games are tearing me apart, and your thoughtless words are breaking my heart. You're breaking my heart." I don't know what attracted him to this song. Was it Jewel's sexy, soulful voice? The harmony? The delicate piano notes with a hint of cello in the background? Or did he somehow relate to the words? I hoped not, but I never understood. "Why do you like this song?" I asked in bewilderment. "I don't know; I just like it," was all he replied.

Caregiving Affirmation:
Don't expect to always understand
why your loved one insists on certain things.

FINALLY, A DIAGNOSIS

Three years and still no diagnosis.

Earlier in the disease, the veteran neurologist at the movement disorders clinic at a Boston hospital had named it "Charles's disease." Now—April 30, 1998—we would meet with the entire staff at this hospital to get an expert opinion. To determine a diagnosis, they would use the progression of symptoms, opinions from other experts such as the neuro-ophthalmologist, and results from PET scans of Charles's brain.

We sat anxiously in the clinic's waiting room, which was filled with patients—some shaking with uncontrollable tremors, others with bodies or limbs cocked in weird positions, and others just staring quietly into space. The neurologist finally retrieved us and led us down a hall to a closed door. As the door opened and I wheeled Charles in, seven doctors in white lab coats stared unemotionally at

us. The room felt dark even though it was sunny and pleasant outside. Was the darkness from the dull fluorescent lighting or from the
heavy sense of gloom I felt?

After introducing us, the neurologist methodically presented
Charles's case to the other doctors. They began asking us questions:
"What were your first symptoms? When did they occur? How did
they progress? How are they affecting Charles now?" His speech slurring, Charles answered the questions, and I helped translate, adding
explanations when necessary. With all of this information to deal
with, the doctors talked out their thought processes, each stressing
some evidence for the diagnosis they were leaning toward.

And then they said it: PSP—progressive supranuclear palsy.

But where was the relief that Charles and I had anticipated feeling? We'd waited three long years for this very moment. To me, it felt
worse having a diagnosis. PSP was the diagnosis I'd expected to hear.
Hope, though, had allowed me to wish for something better.

Caregiving Affirmation:
Prepare yourself for a diagnosis that may be devastating.

After the meeting, Charles and I met alone with this neurologist.
As Charles did at every doctor visit, he asked, "How long do I have to
live?" Until that day, no doctor would pinpoint a realistic time span.
Most doctors responded with a range of years that was very generous.
But that day, this neurologist must have decided to be more honest.
Maybe he felt that with a diagnosis in hand, we deserved a real
answer. And Charles was certainly persistent in wanting to know his
prognosis. The neurologist responded to Charles's pain-filled question: "About five years."

In fact, Charles would live just two more years, but hearing "five
years" sent him into an immediate spiral of depression that he fought
for the remaining months he had left. He would periodically yell out
in frustration, "I only have five years to live!" His hopes of being able
to change the world and make a difference were shattered. Finally
knowing his prognosis deflated his hope and his will to conquer
the disease.

Charles and I left this Boston hospital that day numb with the reality of the news we'd just heard. How eerie it was to watch all the people around us going on with their normal day, as if nothing had happened.

INSPIRATION AND POSITIVE HIGHLIGHTS

OUR CONNECTION TO MORRIE

Tuesdays with Morrie has now become a best-selling book, but it had just been published when Charlie gave a copy to Charles in early 1998.

Charlie, a sociology professor at Boston College, participated with Charles on the steering committee for the college's Leadership for Change graduate-level work-based program. Before joining Boston College, Charlie had worked with Morrie Schwartz more than twenty-five years earlier in Brandeis University's sociology department, and they had remained close friends, seeing each other every week or so over the years. Mitch Albom, the author of *Tuesdays with Morrie*, had interviewed Charlie to add rich details about Morrie's life to his book.

When Charlie handed Charles and me the book at a seventieth birthday party for another Boston College professor, he shared his disappointment that although he'd tried, he never got a chance to introduce Charles to Morrie. Charlie felt they would have identified with each other because of their similar life philosophies—imbedded in their deep caring for other people. But Morrie died without affording that opportunity. Now Charles had developed a degenerative neurological disease similar to Morrie's in its progressive nature. Charlie inscribed in the book he gave to us: "Charles, you share much with Morrie's wisdom. I hope you find his peace and serenity. Love, Charlie." Up to that point, though, Charles hadn't experienced that peace and serenity.

About a year earlier, Charlie had given us a video containing the three TV interviews Morrie gave to Ted Koppel on ABC News's *Nightline*. Charlie believed these would encourage Charles as he faced neurological challenges. But at the time, Charles couldn't watch them.

"Charles, would you like to look at the videos Charlie gave us about Morrie?" I'd ask periodically. He kept refusing. Then one night after we had dinner, I asked again, and to my surprise, he reluctantly replied, "Okay." He dutifully watched the shows, but not with much interest or enthusiasm. I wondered if his resistance came from his fears and wanting to disbelieve that he would be facing similar deterioration—and death. Or maybe Charles couldn't identify because Morrie, in his late seventies at the time of the interviews, was much older than him. He never gave me a concrete reason, but he still made his disinterest clear.

I, on the other hand, found positive messages from Morrie's words that I could repeat back to Charles when I felt the time was right. I'd say, "Like Morrie, Charles, you still have things to offer this world even though the disease is taking away some of your physical capabilities." "Let's be in the moment and go for the quality of life, as Morrie says." "Remember how Morrie indulged his dependence? It's okay to need assistance from others. Helping you provides a way for others to feel valuable." And when Charles would get depressed about his disease's progression, I'd say, "Remember how Morrie would allow himself to cry about his losses? It's okay to be sad and depressed for a little while." Sometimes he would appreciate my encouragement; other times, he'd look at me blankly or ignore me.

Now, though, with the newly published book in hand, Charles gave me permission to read it aloud to him at night before bed. He began to warm up to the concepts behind and comfort of Morrie's words.

And then he watched the video of the *Nightline* interviews again, this time enthusiastically absorbing all the philosophies and encouragement he'd missed the first time around. Was it that enough time had passed for the progression of his disease to be more apparent to him? Or did my encouragement about the messages from Morrie finally sink in? Or maybe just hearing the words from the book allowed him to rethink the messages in the videos.

He asked everyone who visited to watch the video with him. We took it on our trips to visit both of our families and watched it with them. After each viewing, Charles openly and passionately discussed his disease for the first time with all of these people.

Charles drank in all of Morrie's upbeat messages about living while dying—accept your disease, go for things that interest you, be compassionate, be kind to yourself, and don't let the disease diminish your spirit. Morrie's words and his life showed how someone with a terminal illness could still contribute to the world, which encouraged Charles in his mission to make a difference.

But even more than all of those positive messages, Charles seemed to relate the most to Morrie's spiritual search as an agnostic. Morrie never seemed exactly sure of God, but he did come to recognize the contribution his own life made to the world. To him, whatever happened after death would be just fine.

Viewing the video with my "born-again" Christian family prompted some of Charles's most fervent spiritual discussions. Sitting on the ivory leather sofa in my sister Carolyn's house, Charles asked the same questions he'd repeated many times during his searching agnostic years. "Why does God hide himself? Why does a loving God allow suffering?" But now, he really wanted to believe that good answers did exist.

We finished *Tuesdays with Morrie* and then also read Morrie's own book, *Letting Go*. Charles soaked up every word. Morrie's saying

> *Learn how to live, and you'll know how to die;*
> *learn how to die, and you'll know how to live*

most powerfully inspired Charles, allowing him to move on in his disease.

LESSONS FROM MOVIES: DOES THE LOVE END?
"Will you love me for the rest of my life?" he asked, as he lay dying in a hospital bed. "No, I'll love you for the rest of *my* life," she said.

This powerful dialogue came from the movie *Phenomenon* with John Travolta.

Charles loved movies. To him, watching the presentation of the Academy Awards was second only to watching political debates and following presidential elections. Movies enhanced his experiences in life as well as provided him an escape. I soon learned to enjoy them nearly as much as he did. During Charles's illness, I connected in a special way to a couple of movies.

In the movie *Phenomenon*, Travolta's character, George Malley, had a love interest named Lace. Though Lace was interested in George, she didn't let herself fall in love until after it became known that he had an inoperable brain tumor and would soon die. Their moving conversation about how long love lasts came during a touching scene while they snuggled in the hospital. How beautiful to acknowledge that Lace's love would go on, even after George died. I, too, would love Charles for the rest of my life—not just for the rest of his.

In another tender scene, George tried to connect with Lace's two children, around ages eight and ten. The boy was protecting himself from any feelings, presumably to prevent the pain that would come when George died. George shared an analogy using an apple. He said that if he just tossed the apple to the ground and left it there, it would die, spoil, and then be gone in a few days. But if he took a bite from it, the apple would be part of him, and he would then take it with him forever. After a long pause, the little girl and boy took a bite of the apple.

This helped me not to worry about the length of Charles's life and not to hold back my emotions, but to instead experience our relationship to the fullest while we still had time.

Caregiving Affirmation:
Embrace inspirational messages.

UP CLOSE & PERSONAL
"Because You Loved Me" was our theme song.

My sister Barb had just turned on the radio after we situated Charles on the puffy blue sofa in her den. I sat down beside him, with Jack, Barb's husband, sitting across the room, his legs crossed, anticipating an enjoyable conversation.

While had I attended a Blue Cross Blue Shield health promotion conference in Chicago earlier in the day, Charles had spent the time with Barb at her home. Jack and I had caught the train home, arriving early that evening. Barb launched into a description of the adventures earlier in the day.

Barb had arranged to have a home health aide assist with Charles's physical needs during her day alone with him because the effects of a past automobile accident kept Barb from being able to lift or move him. The aide was "sweet but petite," Barb said. "I left for just a few minutes to drive to the grocery store to pick up food for dinner. When I got home, I found Charles sitting on the toilet and the aide pacing around with a panicked look on her face. She confessed that after many grueling attempts, she had not been able to lift Charles off the toilet seat."

"Oh no," I gasped. "I was afraid something like that might happen. How did you finally get him up?"

"We called the police," Barb admitted.

As we all settled in for more conversation, the dynamic voice of Celine Dion began to fill the room. Instantly I recognized that she was on the radio singing our song. Instinctively, I immediately stared straight into Charles's brown eyes, and with tears in mine, I sang along, knowing the words to the chorus by heart. And Charles tried the best he could to also sing with the song, in a hit-or-miss fashion, his eyes fixed on mine.

The first time we'd heard it, Charles and I had known that was our song. "Because You Loved Me" expressed the way we each felt about the other. I truly believed that I was the person I was because of Charles's influence. And I think he felt the same toward me. Though we fell in love with the song when we heard it on the radio, we later learned that it was the theme song for the movie *Up Close & Personal*. I soon discovered that the story of the movie also seemed to parallel our life together.

Tally Atwater, played by Michelle Pfeiffer, wanted to be a television reporter. Warren Justice, a successful TV news producer played by Robert Redford, saw her potential and hired her. Over time, Warren taught her how to be a good reporter—not just reporting the facts, but listening to people and reporting the human story beneath the facts. Warren coached her and helped her become the best reporter, drawing on her inner resources. They eventually married.

After a while, Warren realized that Tally had learned how to be a great, caring reporter—he had taught her well. He then decided to follow through on some of his own personal goals and took an assignment in Panama—and was killed. Tally was able to go on—and become a network anchor—because of the foundation, coaching, love, and support that Warren had given.

In a similar way, Charles's unconditional love gave me the self-esteem I needed to find my potential and thrive. He helped me to grow tremendously as a person and a professional. He helped me become a better writer, a more polished public speaker, and a respected leader. He helped me blossom into a better person. I am everything I am because Charles loved me. Even though he would die young, his life would live on through me.

As this moment played out in Barb's den, I became only peripherally aware that Barb and Jack, also with eyes full of tears, observed the tender connection between Charles and me.

Living Life to Its Fullest

Washington, D.C., Austin, Atlanta, and Russia—we visited plenty of places in that year of rapid physical decline for Charles. And when not traveling, he continued to participate in the activities he found meaningful. Throughout, I found serenity in seeing Charles meet his goals and do things that fed his self-worth.

Attending His Last ESOP Events

The ESOP board of directors held its semiannual meeting in Austin, Texas, early that year. I suggested that maybe he could see his friend Randall while we were there. Randall and Charles had been very good friends in college, so Charles was excited about their getting together again.

Randall arrived in his Toyota Camry to pick up Charles at the hotel. I gave him some quick instructions on how to care for Charles's needs, and they took off to his apartment. I'm sure that Randall struggled with understanding Charles, who now couldn't always put his thoughts together or articulate them clearly, but neither of these longtime friends wanted to miss an opportunity for a reunion.

✦✦✦✦✦

A few months later, the director of the ESOP Association stunned Charles and me when he called us at home and said, "The board of trustees for the Employee Ownership Foundation has decided to start a scholarship in Charles's honor. The scholarship would allow nonmanagement employees of employee-owned companies to win one thousand dollars toward reimbursement of a training program or conference. We'll give out two this year. We've decided to call them the Charles R. Edmunson Scholarships."

"Wow, Charles," I said after hanging up the phone. "They've created a scholarship in your name! That will be there long after you and I are gone. What a legacy!"

"Yeah," Charles said, with a perplexed smile on his face.

Usually that kind of honor comes after the person has died. I hoped that Charles could understand its significance and fully experience the pleasure of this tribute while he was still alive.

Meanwhile, two of Charles's colleagues from the ESOP Association, Steve and Ginny, had invited him to participate in their presentation at one of the sessions to be held at the annual conference in May. I thought, *Are they crazy? Steve* (who had accompanied Charles on the trip to Hungary) *should know that Charles struggles to express his thoughts. How can Charles possibly contribute and not embarrass himself?* Then an idea popped into my head.

"Charles," I said, "why don't we prepare your speech in writing before you go? That way, if you have a hard time expressing your thoughts and grabbing your words, Ginny, Steve, or I could read it."

"Okay, that sounds good," he replied, appearing as relieved as I was to have this alternative. As we prepared the piece, we focused on the messages from his book, *Paradoxes of Leadership*. This would be the only time Charles got to present these principles to an audience.

Attending the conference had its share of difficulties. The shower at the hotel, though a walk-in, had a funny slant to it, and a lip. When I tried to maneuver the shower hose and keep contact with Charles, he tumbled off the shower chair and onto the floor, with me holding onto him to break his fall. Faced with a soaking-wet Charles and a slippery shower floor, I had to call the front desk for help. Someone there called the police, who not only helped pick up Charles but also assisted me in finishing his shower and getting him dressed in his light blue shirt and navy blue sport coat.

The presentation with Ginny and Steve went well. Then that evening, the awards banquet sparkled with excitement. Near the end of the ceremony, the president of the ESOP Association, Michael, surprised us again not only by awarding the actual scholarships to the winners, but also by presenting them with a hardcover copy of the tribute book that Charles's friends had given him the previous year. Michael had written an introduction to the book, which he read aloud to the audience:

> *As a recipient of the Charles R. Edmunson Scholarship from the Employee Ownership Foundation, the Foundation and its employee owner supporters want you to have this book that pays tribute to the man for whom the scholarship is named.*
>
> *We ask that in the next few days and months, you take the time to read the wonderful tributes to the man who has probably done more to make employee ownership a moving and real experience for his colleagues at the company where he worked, Web Industries, Inc., and for so many other individuals from across America, who shared with him a vision for America of self-worth, maximized human potential, and respect for other people, ideas, and for all human emotions.*
>
> *We believe that these tributes will inspire you to reach, even if a little more, to conduct your life as someone who reaches out to individuals, and who in doing so embodies those qualities that Charles has taught so many employee owners—those qualities that can make a difference in America, and even the world.*
>
> *Treasure these words of tribute to Charles, as we who know Charles cherish his life work for employee ownership.*

After the ceremony, Charles stared up into space, not able to focus his eyes on the people around him. But the wide smile on his face gave away his feeling of awe. The two scholarship recipients held his hands and told him how much they had admired him while I signed their copy of the tribute book on his behalf.

SUPPORTING THE EMPLOYEES AT FRAMINGHAM

The entire workforce at the Web Converting plant in Framingham gathered to attend a two-day program by a motivational trainer on teamwork and improving work processes, an unprecedented event for the plant. Machine operators, secretaries, support staff—everyone would be attending. Charles was determined to participate and encourage the employees in learning new and much-needed skills.

Unfortunately, the conference room at the old plant was on the second floor, and there was no elevator. The employees, though, had already figured out how they would get Charles up there. They loaded him in his wheelchair and onto a forklift, raised him up to the second level, and unloaded him there, just like they would do for their manufacturing materials.

During the program, Charles found a few ways to share his thoughts to encourage the employees and managers to take the training to heart, but it wasn't easy for him. When he talked, his speech slurred and was difficult for some to understand, frustrating him. And because the restroom was a few steps down on another level, when Charles needed to go to the bathroom, we took him into an adjacent conference room to have him urinate into the plastic cup. At the time, Charles also struggled with gas. He couldn't control himself—he just let go, putting him in an embarrassing situation. Nonetheless, he was determined to be a part of this unique training for the employees at the plant he loved so much.

HOSTING A NEIGHBORHOOD PARTY

We were the new ones in the neighborhood. But from what I could figure out, very few of the neighbors knew each other. I wanted to feel connected with other people because my connection with Charles was slowly being severed. And I figured that if I wanted this, I would have to initiate it.

On one of my walks up our mile-long street, I jotted down the numbers from the mailboxes for all the houses. On the party invitations I purchased, I addressed the envelopes to "Neighbor" and then put in each house's street address, city, and zip code. Inside, I wrote that this was an invitation to attend a neighborhood get-together. I had no idea if anyone would come. To my surprise, nearly half of the neighbors called to let me know they would attend.

With Charles now in a wheelchair and getting uncomfortable and irritable quickly, I started to wonder if I could pull this party off. How would I greet the guests, keep the food and drinks refreshed, and carry on the conversations I yearned for?

As I described earlier, in answer to my dilemma, my sister Sue from West Virginia called. "Janet, I want to come and visit some time. When would be good for you?"

"What perfect timing," I said, delighted. "I'm panicking about how I am going to host a neighborhood party in two weeks. Do you think you could come that weekend?"

Sue and her daughter, Rachel, made it all work. Charles and I greeted the guests at the door. Some of the neighbors would have seen me pushing Charles up and down the street in his wheelchair before the party, but I know that others were a bit shocked to see him for the first time. And he did require my constant attention during the party to keep him occupied.

Sue and Rachel kept the food and drinks going. And after all arrived, I enjoyed finding out which house people lived in, what they did for a living, how many kids they had, and other tidbits of information. The party sparked more neighborhood events, including regular women's nights out and an annual neighborhood holiday party. A real sense of community began to develop.

Caregiving Affirmation:
Live life to the fullest at every opportunity.

AND WE'RE OFF TO RUSSIA!

Mom did it again.

In the fall of 1997, Charles and I were sitting comfortably in the living room of our newly rented apartment when Mom called. During our conversation, she said, "Some of my friends are planning to go on a trip to Russia. I'm thinking about joining them. What do you think?"

Without hesitation, Charles said, "I want to go." I knew immediately that I had no choice—we would be going to Russia. I didn't know whether by the time of the trip—about eight months after the initial registration—he would be physically capable of going. His quick deterioration had already caused us to move from our wonderful Victorian home into this apartment before our new house was ready, so I really wanted us to stay home. But he argued that he had always wanted to visit Russia. In getting his master's degree in philosophy, he wrote his dissertation on the ethical roots of Marxism. Just before we had moved into the apartment, he had asked me to look for his dissertation in our dusty old metal file cabinets. I had started reading it aloud to him in the evenings before bed. What timing Mom had! Charles was determined to go, no matter what the obstacles.

Marcia, the travel agent for the trip, had coordinated and led it a number of times in the past. In talking with her to set up our registration, I soon learned of the difficulties we would face.

We would be traveling by ship, starting in St. Petersburg and then proceeding down the river and lake system in Russia, ending in Moscow. The ship was *not* a luxury cruise liner, Marcia advised: Each tiny cabin's bathroom doubled as a shower. Marcia told me that I would have to put the toilet seat down and close the curtain around the entire space. "This might actually be helpful for Charles," she said, "as he could sit on the toilet seat when showering." What I didn't know was how tight the space really was, how difficult it would be for me to get Charles up and down from the toilet seat, and how unsteady he would be while sitting on the toilet with nothing to hold on to during the shower.

The next fear centered on how we would be able to get Charles on and off, as well as around, the ship. The ship offered no bedrooms on the floor where the dining hall was located. That meant stair climbing, because the ship didn't have an elevator. And our room would be one level down from the exit level—requiring more climbing. In addition, the function rooms, where the lectures were conducted, were on yet another level—two stories up! When we registered for the trip, Charles was still walking with assistance and didn't have a wheelchair—but stairs were quickly becoming impossible.

And then there would be the long airplane flight. Charles's incontinence would require some creative solutions. Could he even tolerate sitting on the plane for that long?

Why would I even agree to this trip with these known obstacles—let alone the ones I feared but hadn't yet discovered? I knew that to him, this was a dream come true. How could I say no? He was dying and his body was degenerating. More deterioration was inevitable, but I had to take the chance. I had committed myself to giving Charles the best experiences possible despite his disease. I had to give it a try.

⁂

By the time of the trip, Charles was using a wheelchair most of the time. He struggled desperately to get sleep, and his incontinence continued. These issues provided the foundation for most of our struggles throughout the trip.

I decided to invite someone, in addition to my mother, who could help us. I knew that Cal, who had worked at the Framingham plant, would enjoy Russia because he had a fondness for Lenin's values. He gladly accepted my invitation. The trip turned out to be the beginning of Cal's love of the Russian people. He has since returned to Russia at least four times.

Cal provided tremendous help to us. He came to the rescue at the times when Charles was stuck on the toilet because I couldn't get him up. He helped with the daily needs of getting Charles dressed, wheeling him around the unforgiving Russian streets, and staying with Charles at times so I could see the sights. We were fortunate that my sister and brother-in-law, Barb and Jack, could also go on the trip. Between all of us—and it often *did* take all of us—we got Charles around Russia.

The biggest group effort was getting Charles up and down the ship stairs. I would often tip the Russian sailors, and they would carry Charles up the stairs in his wheelchair. But they weren't always around. So Cal and Jack would take Charles's arms, standing at his side. Barb and I would be behind at Charles's feet. Mom would hold all the gear. On each step, the guys would stabilize and lift Charles up to the next step while Barb would lift and steady the first foot. Once that was clearly in place, I would lift and steady the second foot. One foot at a time, we'd painstakingly work our way up the stairs. By the end of the vacation, unfortunately, both Cal and Jack had strained their backs!

Later, when asked what his favorite part of the trip was, Charles always commented on how nice the Russian people were. A person in a wheelchair was an uncommon sight in Russia. *Babushkas*—poor elderly women typically wearing a scarf around their head—would put the wildflowers they were selling to tourists for one dollar in Charles's lap to show how touched they were by his misfortune.

Another highlight for Charles was quite unexpected. He and Cal paused in amazement as Sev, the wonderful lecturer on the boat, mentioned employee ownership—Charles's passion—in one of his talks. Charles believed that every worker should have a stake in the profits of the company—and more importantly, that every worker should be valued and respected as an owner. We later met alone with Sev to talk about how he'd learned about employee ownership and his thoughts about the difficulties in making it work in Russia. The good fortune of having Sev as our lecturer gave the trip a deeper meaning for Charles and Cal.

Despite all of the positive elements, Charles didn't seem to fully enjoy the trip as he had earlier ones; he couldn't move his eyes appropriately to see everything. And his brain, at this point in the disease, had already started to impede his thought processes.

On the other hand, for me, this trip not only provided a wonderfully touching experience with Charles, Cal, and my family, but also revealed a very different and special culture. I thoroughly enjoyed taking in all of the famous sights—the tremendously opulent mansions, museums with classical works of art, churches with elaborate icons, the infamous Kremlin and Red Square, and Lenin embalmed in his tomb.

Somehow, I found the everyday lives of ordinary people the most poignant part of our trip. We happened upon a wedding party at one of the monasteries, a line of babushkas selling vegetables on the street, a day care center where the children still used chamber pots because of the lack of plumbing, and the colorful markets where the Russians shopped.

But as I'd feared, the practical difficulties of traveling were real—and even greater than we had expected.

Charles and I had traveled enough recently for me to know that the airplane ride would be a challenge. His body would stiffen, making the tight space and uncomfortable seats nearly unbearable. And the airplane restrooms would be impossible. On past trips, I'd strained to stuff the two of us in the tiny airplane bathroom and shut the door, where I'd undress and assist him. His capabilities had declined tremendously since the last trip, and I knew for certain that I couldn't handle this, nor could Cal.

So despite our past bad experiences with condom catheters, on this trip I decided to try one that strapped to Charles's leg and had a valve to make sure that the urine would travel effectively to the catheter bag. This was different enough from what we'd used before that I was anxious about what would happen if it didn't work. Finding out on the plane would be too late!

Well, my fears were realized when urine started to leak onto his clothes. We had to go into the tiny restroom on the airplane after all. At the time, I didn't know if the leak was caused by putting the contraption on incorrectly, or by a hole in the catheter. "Why do I have to wear this?" Charles complained, while Cal assisted me in changing Charles's clothes and catheter. I was relieved to discover that the source of the problem was indeed a hole in the condom and not a malfunction of the entire catheter.

But that wasn't the only challenge that Charles's incontinence provided. It was impossible to make sure that a restroom would be available whenever he needed one in Russia. So we brought along a urinal and had him use that on the bus after everyone disembarked. This not only embarrassed Charles but also made it difficult for us to get the timing right.

Charles's body never adjusted to the new time zone. Even the sleeping pills were useless. He ended up sleeping during the day on the bus and being wide awake all night. The only way for me to survive and get at least some sleep was to put Charles's cassette player and headphones on him to keep him occupied. The tape player had automatic reverse, but the tapes still needed to be changed every ninety minutes to two hours. Just as at home, my exhaustion from lack of sleep mounted.

Transporting Charles was difficult throughout the trip because Russia is not handicapped-accessible. In the one museum that did have an elevator, visitors needed special permission to use it, which wasn't easy to obtain. And the one handicapped-accessible stall we found in a restroom was padlocked. (I now appreciate tremendously the work of the disabled and their advocates in the United States for laws that have made accessibility a right.)

The plane trip home was even tougher than the trip over. Fortunately, the condom catheter worked. But Charles's lack of sleep and increasing stiffness made the return trip physically intolerable. Cal and I were constantly trying to comfort and calm him. We'd take him for walks down the aisles, but to no avail. At one point, Charles insisted in all seriousness, "Stop the plane. I want to get off!"

The trip took a real toll on Charles's health. He didn't bounce back physically when we returned, but instead, his deterioration seemed to almost accelerate from that weakened point. Nevertheless, going to Russia offered Charles the opportunity to reach yet another personal goal and to have a new experience. Attaining that goal was as important to him as actually going on the trip.

Many of the forty people in the tour group commented on how they were touched to see the care my family, Cal, and I gave Charles. I hoped that our example would be an inspiration to the new friends we had met.

And the trip brought me amazing memories that were well worth the huge effort. I would do it again—even knowing the extreme difficulties we would face. My life is richer for the struggle and accomplishment of that adventure. The alternative—not going on the trip and just watching Charles deteriorate at home—would have been far worse.

Saying Good-bye in Atlanta

The picture still makes me giggle.

Charles and I combined a Labor Day family reunion in Atlanta with a visit to the Web Converting plant there that he had managed in the 1980s. I don't think Charles realized it, but I knew that this would be the last time for the employees there to see the leader they so dearly loved. Though the words were never said, I was giving them a chance to say good-bye.

I wheeled Charles into the conference room at the plant that he had helped build, and one by one, the employees came in to talk to him. Some had accents from India, others from Laos; the rest were Southern. Charles would often look at them in bewilderment but at precious times would crack a big smile or laugh. It was hard to know how much he was absorbing. But the words from each employee, while mostly in broken English, must have touched his heartstrings.

After that emotional visit, we returned to my brother's house for our weekend family activities—picnicking and watching the laser show at Stone Mountain State Park, enjoying spaghetti made for the masses of family, and just catching up.

My artsy nephew, Evan, who always had a cutting-edge—and sometimes weird—hairstyle, was wearing his hair spiked. (Though the style isn't so unusual now, it was then.) With the help of lots of mousse, the short ends stood straight up—dark at the roots and bleached blond on the tips.

The "uncles," my brother and brothers-in-law, conspired to look the same as Evan—and they included Charles in the shenanigans. While none of them looked as sharp as Evan did, Doug's thick hair did the best. Tony and Curt looked silly, but not nearly as ridiculous as Jack, whose deeply receding hairline allowed a few meager strands of hair, about five inches long, to stand straight up, like Alfalfa in *The Little Rascals*.

I roared loudest, however, when I looked at Charles. My brother Doug caught just the right moment with his camera. Laughing out loud, I was pushing Charles in his wheelchair into public view. With sunglasses, spiked hair, and a totally blank expression on his face, he looked like one of the Blues Brothers being cool. As soon as we lined up all of the men with their new hairdos for the group picture, Charles's blank look erupted into his gorgeous smile, clearly showing his willingness to join in the fun.

After the reunion, Doug combined that picture with others in one of those collage frames that display a half dozen or so pictures. I hung it on the wall in front of the treadmill I used everyday. Throughout the rest of Charles's life—when his diseased brain took away so much, including his ability to laugh—seeing this picture would always make me chuckle, giving me the comic relief I so badly needed.

NOT TAKING CARE OF ME

From the time we woke up until the time we went to bed, every minute was filled—jogging with Charles, getting myself showered and dressed, going to work, having dinner and our frozen yogurt, then getting Charles ready for bed. During the week, we at least had the aides in the morning, at work, and in the early evenings. But on the weekends, I was all alone with Charles. When was there time for taking care of me?

This had been the most difficult year of Charles's disease so far. Physically and emotionally, I had been focusing solely on him, not me. And with our sleep deprivation, that was all I had the energy to do. I longed to have some mental breaks, my own exercise routine, enough sleep each night, and time to go to dinner or a movie with friends. I pressed on, however, not allowing my needs and emotions to interfere with what I had to do.

And Charles never asked about how I was doing. I suspect he wasn't capable of being curious about my feelings. Early in the disease, it might have been because he was the one facing all of the losses. Now I wasn't sure that he could express any concerns for me even if he felt them—and I didn't expect him to. Before the disease, he had always taken care of my needs. Now the circumstances were just too overwhelming for him.

When I went shopping for some much-needed new suits for work,

I was aghast that I had jumped up one dress size—and was teetering on the edge of going up one more. I was sure the extra pounds were caused by my now-minimal exercise routine—creeping along at a snail's pace with Charles and not having time to go for my own run. And I'm sure that satisfying my sweet tooth, one of my few remaining simple pleasures, was also to blame.

The caregiving also caused me physical wear and tear. All of the buttoning and unbuttoning, zipping and unzipping, lifting pants on and pulling them off that I had done for Charles accelerated the development of arthritis in my thumbs. I could now hardly open a jar. My only relief came from occasionally taking a quick minute at the end of the day to circle my thumbs in a bowl of hot water with Epsom salts.

Going to work each day provided me with a sense of normalcy amidst the turmoil at home. But it gave me no emotional reprieve from the chaos that my life had become.

All of the professionals—the doctors, nurses, and health agency representatives—as well as friends and family told us, the caregivers, to take care of ourselves. While we consciously knew we needed to do it, actually fulfilling our own needs seemed next to impossible. I had six of the ten warning signs of caregiver stress listed in the Alzheimer's Association brochure—anxiety, exhaustion, sleeplessness, irritability, lack of concentration, and health problems. (The other four are denial, anger, social withdrawal, and depression.)

I guess I thought I was young and could handle it—and somehow, I was getting by. But the reality was that I had to spend so much energy on Charles's day-to-day needs that I couldn't come up with creative solutions that would support my own needs. Caring for myself had become much more challenging than caring for Charles.

Caregiving Affirmation:
Watch for the warning signs of caregiver stress.

BIG FINISH TO THE YEAR

WHEN THE YELLING STARTED

In November, we were back in the hospital again—only one week after a four-day stay in which Dr. Ravin conducted a trial on Charles for a baclofen pump. Each of the four days, Dr. Ravin injected the drug baclofen directly into Charles's spinal cord. If the drug worked, he would find his rigid muscles loosening, allowing him to walk more easily, though still with assistance. And he would then be a candidate to have a pump inserted into his body that would release just the right amount of the drug to give him relief.

During the first day of the trial, we thought he experienced some improvement. But as each day progressed, the gains stopped. By the end of the four days, Dr. Ravin disappointed both of us and, I think, herself, by admitting, "The trial just didn't work. We should have seen more response to the drug. We won't be able to insert the pump."

During the hospital stay, though, Charles seemed to do fine emotionally. For the most part, he remained tolerant of the procedures. Deedee came each day to help with his needs, and Darry and I attended to him each evening. I spent the nights with Charles, sleeping in a reclining chair next to his bed.

Then after being back at home for only one week, Charles scared Darry with a bout of shortness of breath. Before I got home from work, Darry had called 911, and the ambulance had whisked Charles off to UMass Memorial Medical Center again. A hospital room became our home for another four days.

Luckily, Deedee and Darry continued to come to the hospital during their normal shifts and provided the personal care and attention the hospital staff just couldn't give. Without them, Charles could have been ignored more than other patients because he couldn't clearly communicate his needs or help himself in any way.

The shortness of breath went away on its own on the first evening, and he started to do much better. But the hospital staff members wouldn't let Charles go home until they had completed numerous tests. We felt stuck there.

The cardiac enzymes test results were negative—so he hadn't had a heart attack. Even so, the doctors ordered an echocardiogram and a thallium stress electrocardiogram. Typically the stress test is performed on a treadmill. For Charles, who couldn't stand or walk on his own, the chemical method would have to be used. The chemical he was injected with simulated physical stress on his heart, allowing the radioactive isotope thallium to show where his heart wasn't performing well. I worried that Charles wouldn't be able to lie still during the test, but all went reasonably well.

Once complete, though, the test didn't show us anything new. And what would we have done if it had? I'm not sure I would have wanted Charles to take cardiac medications again. He already had a complicated regimen of medications for his neurological condition. He had faithfully committed to eating a low-fat diet. I pondered whether at that point, a fatal heart attack would have been merciful for him.

The pulmonologist checked his lung function, and the speech pathologist conducted a barium swallow. Both showed minor problems, but nothing that could be treated.

I don't know why, but I agreed to let them give Charles a sleep test one night. I suspected that Charles had sleep apnea, which is a potentially life-threatening condition that causes numerous night-time episodes of breath-holding and then gasping to take in oxygen.

He'd had that problem in his late thirties, and his doctor had suggested that he take a sleep test—but his hectic schedule got in the way. When he later lost weight, the symptoms went away. Earlier in the neurodegenerative disease, though, it had started again—holding his breath and then gasping for air in the deepest part of his sleep. I thought the problem might be caused by his latest antidepressant, doxepin. But at that point, what good would it be for us to officially know that he had sleep apnea? He probably wouldn't have tolerated any of the treatments for it, the most common one entailing wearing a mask over the face while sleeping.

During the sleep test, the technician carefully attached electrodes all over Charles's head and body. He struggled to lie still. I suspected from the way he cringed and looked panicked that the technicians would struggle to get clear results. And I was right. Charles's agitation did not allow him to sleep enough for them to get valid results. This was just another test that aggravated Charles.

As each day progressed, his emotional stability deteriorated. He seemed exasperated from being cooped up in the sterile white-and-chrome hospital room. Then he started yelling. At the top of his lungs, he screamed, "Ahhhhhhh!"

Charles tried to tell us what was bothering him. I desperately tried to understand what he said, but most of the time, with his badly slurred speech, I just couldn't. Feeling even more frustrated, he'd yell, "Ahhhhhhh!" Nothing appeased him except the occasional frozen yogurt Darry brought him.

Maybe he was trying to tell us that he wanted to go home. And why should he continue to stay? His symptoms improved after the first twenty-four hours. The other tests didn't appear to me to be necessary. But Charles presented an intriguing case for the residents.

By that point, Charles was yelling almost constantly. I tried to persuade him that his yelling would disturb his hospital roommate. But he didn't seem to care—or understand. Nothing we tried seemed to help. Each yell disturbed my peace, frustrating me and wearing down my patience. And I felt embarrassed, not being able to control Charles in a public environment.

Fortunately, Dr. Ravin witnessed his yelling on her hospital rounds. Compassionately, she said to me outside the room, "I want to prescribe a new drug, Seroquel. I think it will help with the yelling. We'll start him on twenty-five milligrams two times a day." Oh, what a miracle drug that turned out to be—but only months later, we had to increase the dose and give it to him four times a day.

MORE EPISODES

The next week after leaving the hospital, Charles and I had our traditional Thanksgiving supper with his good friend June and her circle of friends. We'd maintained that custom for a few years. The dinners generally grew into thoughtful, intense discussions about life, politics, and world events. But not that year.

My first concern was how we would get Charles into the house, which had stairs no matter which way you entered. Neighbors came by and, in the pouring rain, lifted Charles in his wheelchair up to the porch so we could wheel him in. Enjoying turkey, mashed potatoes, sweet potatoes, green beans, and cranberry sauce, Charles made it through the dinner just fine. But then as dessert started, his agitation began to simmer, and before long, he started yelling, in front of everyone. We quickly summoned the neighbors again for their assistance, and then left.

On the Saturday night of that Thanksgiving weekend, Charles and I had reservations, made quite some time earlier, to spend the night at the luxurious Charles Hotel in Cambridge. The New England ESOP Association had given us this treat in gratitude for his service as its president for many years. I had invited June and a few other ESOP friends to join us for dinner that evening. Crossing my fingers, I hoped our luck had changed. Could Charles make it through the dinner without yelling?

Shortly after the beautifully arranged pasta meals had been served, Charles started. I repositioned him, talked to him, cajoled him, and did everything I could think of to make him comfortable and quiet down. But it didn't work. Because he was disturbing others in the restaurant, I wheeled him outside while our friends finished their dinner.

Next on the agenda that night was a trip to a pub that had a band performing Beatles songs. I felt sure he would find pleasure in satisfying his Beatles obsession by listening to a live band. Our friends rejoined us and seemed willing to try again to redeem the evening.

We grabbed a taxi and traveled a few miles to the pub. "I Want to Hold Your Hand," "She Loves You, Yeah, Yeah, Yeah," and "Hard Day's Night" rang through the small, crowded pub, the band sounding just like the Beatles. Charles enjoyed the concert but teetered on agitation throughout. When we got him back safely to our hotel room, the yelling started again. June tried to calm him, but she had little success, and quickly grew as frustrated as I had been. Throughout the night, Charles struggled to find his peace and only slept fitfully. Our special night in this wonderful hotel didn't live up to my hopes and probably unreasonable expectations.

Wanting to keep life as normal as possible, I continued to take Charles to his favorite breakfast restaurant on the weekends— Sunnyside Café in Ashland. He loved this outing. Surely we could continue this tradition, I hoped. As he sat in his wheelchair at the wooden table in the middle of the restaurant, I ordered his regular pancakes with cranberries and nuts, along with a fruit cup. Unfortunately, this visit would be our last. Partway through our breakfast, Charles started to yell.

For me, each difficult experience built on the frustration of the last. Did this mean that I couldn't take Charles out anymore? Was his ability to socialize outside of the house gone?

His yelling continued off and on at home. At first I thought it was directed at me: Was it his frustration that I couldn't understand what he said? Was I not keeping him comfortable enough? Or was it that I simply didn't understand what he needed? Or could it be that I was just introducing too many things he found unpleasant—a urinal, Depends pads, nightly condom catheters, a wheelchair?

I took it so personally that one night, in the midst of one of Charles's yelling episodes, I finally lost it. I looked him straight in the eyes and then yelled back at him. "Ehhhhhhh!" I cried, for as long as I had breath. Then at the top of my lungs, I screamed, "How do you like that? Would you like me to yell at you just like you yell at me?" Then, horrified at what I had done, I began sobbing and begged for forgiveness. Too concerned about my loss of control, I don't remember whether Charles stopped yelling in surprise at my actions or whether he instead kept his same demeanor. But I never did that again. It was one of my very lowest points in caring for Charles.

WHAT COULD BE CAUSING THIS? WHAT WOULD HELP?

I could count on one hand the times I had heard Charles yell in all the years we were married. He was such a caring, sensitive person, always willing to compromise. He could articulately share his feelings. He didn't need to yell. So the yelling he was doing at this point must have definitely been a manifestation of the disease. His disease had started to affect his inner as well as his outer self—changing his personality.

As the yelling continued, I began to wonder if it sprang from his physical discomfort. His body remained stiff all the time. With lack of sleep, he must have been continually exhausted. He struggled with incontinence and bowel movements. All of these were perfectly good reasons to make anyone want to yell in frustration.

And he also faced some very difficult transitions in his life, most notably preparing to retire and live at home. Charles had always said he would never retire. I remember many conversations while he was still healthy where he insisted, "I want to work for the rest of my life. Work provides the laboratory for me to impact others."

Just recently, the founder of the company, Bob (now semiretired himself), had coaxed Charles to voluntarily retire before Web would have to ask him to. I knew that Charles's contributions at work had become extremely limited—and his disease made sitting in the office nearly unbearable. We eventually met with the management team at Web and discussed the inevitable. Charles came home feeling totally dejected. Could the likely causes of some of these outbursts be his frustration, fears, and anxiety at accepting retirement and being confined to home?

One day I noticed that he looked different when he yelled. His eyes revealed a deep fear. After his next panicked yell, I asked him, "Charles, is something scaring you?" He clearly replied, "Yes," his eyes beseeching me for help. Lately he'd been confusing yes and no, but not this time. Putting the pieces of the puzzle together, I realized that some of the yelling might be coming from hallucinations— maybe from the disease, or possibly from the medications he took. It helped me a bit to know that perhaps the yelling was not solely due to frustration with me.

The yelling affected not only me but also the aides—especially Deedee, who was with Charles the most. It took her quite a while to tell me that she couldn't stand it anymore. She hated to ever admit that she struggled with caring for Charles. When she finally said something to me, she was on the verge of quitting.

COULD I KEEP HIM AT HOME?

"You'll probably put me in a nursing home," Charles had said back in 1996, lashing out in frustration when he recognized how dependent he was on me for his daily needs. Behind that accusation, I'm sure, was his fear of someday being transplanted from a familiar, comfortable environment to a sterile, unfamiliar one.

Sitting next to him on the love seat in the kitchen sitting area, I reassured him, without hesitation, that I would not put him in a nursing home. I promised to keep him home no matter what happened. I was confident that we would have the financial means to do so. I hadn't thought of the emotional energy that might also be required.

In the early stages of this disease, this pledge provided the foundation for our actions. I was committed to doing whatever it would take to provide for Charles's needs at work and at home. I reassured him that he didn't need to worry—even though I know he still did. I was sure that I wouldn't consider a nursing home as an option.

But now with the overwhelming frustration of his constant yelling, could I still keep that promise? Extremely disappointed, I had to admit to myself that maybe I couldn't. Charles's persistent yelling eroded my can-do attitude and created tremendous inner turmoil. Nothing I or the aides tried seemed to alleviate the cause of his emotional or physical pain—and therefore the yelling. I imagined that it was much like having a colicky baby. The baby continues to cry even when you've fed, cleaned, and cuddled it. That was the worst frustration of all—not being able to do anything to make the situation better.

After Charles died, I listened to a caregiver cassette tape that my brother-in-law Jack had obtained for us from his company's EAP. It provided terrific advice through real-life interviews with caregivers. One of the interviews was with a man who took care of his wife who suffered from a degenerative disease. She wanted him to promise to never put her in a nursing home. He clearly told her that he couldn't make that guarantee because he couldn't predict what her needs might be in the future, and whether he would be capable of meeting them. The experts on the tape agreed that caregivers should always keep the door open, as circumstances can change. It is true that we can't predict the challenges to come—but in my case, I still don't think I would have made a different decision.

I also was still young and healthy. I could continue to physically care for Charles, and our financial situation would allow us to get the help we needed in the home. The freedom of this choice isn't available to everyone, but I'm confident that keeping him home was the right decision for us.

CHRISTMAS ADVENTURES

Music surrounded us. The choir members, in white robes with gold trim, filed in from the sides and circled to the rear, then walked straight down the center to the front of historic Trinity Church in Boston. We had great seats on the right side near the front. Because Charles traveled in a wheelchair, we had entered the church through the handicapped entrance, ahead of the long lines waiting outside in the cold to enter and see one of the most acclaimed Christmas concerts in Boston.

It took John and his son Josh, both strong and over six feet tall, to place Charles's stiff body into the wooden pew. Going to the Trinity Church Christmas concert with the Duncans was becoming a ritual for us. And this year, the music fully engaged us with its intensity and grace. Charles remained peaceful throughout the concert, his eyes and smile sparkling; he seemed to enjoy the Christmas spirit the event revived in him.

But then we pushed our luck a little too far. After the concert, we had dinner with the Duncans at our special restaurant, TGI Friday's on Exeter Street, where Charles and I had spent many nights flirting when we first dated. But now Charles didn't join in the conversation much at all. The disease had inhibited his thought processes, and his struggle to articulate made it impossible to understand when he did venture to say something. Just before dessert was served, he had had enough. "Ahhhhhhh," he yelled, signifying his discomfort and his need to move on. Knowing that the yelling would only intensify, we scurried to finish and get him out before his escalating yells would disturb the entire restaurant.

A few weeks later, Mom visited, and the two of us took Charles to the Boston Pops Christmas concert. We wheeled Charles into Symphony Hall next to one of the small tables in the auditorium. Charles stayed in his wheelchair while Mom and I sat in the white, wooden folding chairs around the little table.

But Charles's brain kept giving his body the wrong signals. It should have been telling some muscles to contract and the opposing muscles to relax. Instead, his brain's messages kept all muscles contracted. So during the concert, after I had pushed hard to keep his feet on the footrests of the wheelchair and his rear end snugly into the seat, his body would slowly stiffen—which meant his legs would straighten, his feet would slide off the footrests, and his entire body would slide off the seat of his wheelchair. To get him back in place, I had to get in front of him, lift him to a standing position, ease him back into the chair, and then push his feet back to place them on the footrests. (This was before I had the "aha" moment that led me to strap his feet to the footrests with a cloth belt.)

The first time I attempted to reposition him during the concert, his feet slipped on the slick wooden floor of the auditorium when I lifted him to a stand. No matter how I tried, and even with Mom's assistance, I couldn't get Charles situated back into his wheelchair. Before he slipped totally onto the floor, which had happened before at home, I needed to wheel him out to the foyer where there was a carpeted floor. Between songs I pushed him out to reposition him, and then before the next song, I wheeled him back in. He'd last for a song or two and then slowly stiffen again and begin slithering off his seat.

We made it through the concert, but not without disturbing the audience a number of times. The physical effort and emotional results of all this tested me almost more than I could handle—but not quite. Nonetheless, Mom and I still found the concert moving, glad to have had the opportunity to experience this type of special holiday entertainment. But in contrast to the Trinity Church event, Charles couldn't feel the peace and delight of the evening because his discomfort got in the way.

Just before Christmas, more of my family arrived. My sister Barb came from Chicago with her husband, Jack, and Carolyn arrived from Florida with her husband and two children. Both families didn't want Charles and me to be alone for the holidays. Because Charles could no longer travel, we were stuck at home. We all had a special time together. But at that point, his yelling wasn't yet controlled by the Seroquel, and I didn't yet fully understand the causes. I wish I had been more resourceful at the time in dealing with it. Being with others—even family members—when he yelled intensified my frustration and embarrassment. And I know it disturbed them, too.

In the midst of these trying circumstances, I was preparing to host a PSP support group meeting in January. After sending out the invitations, I received a call from the wife of a man who had recently died from PSP. She told me that she wouldn't be able to attend the meeting but wanted me to pass her name and phone number on to others. "They should all feel free to call me," she said. "I might be able to answer some of their questions." The woman spoke very freely to me about her husband, his disease, his life, and his death. I felt safe in asking her about their decision on nursing homes. She described a terrifying experience:

> *When my husband's disease was quite advanced, he got sick and developed pneumonia. We needed to admit him into the hospital. I realized at this point that I might not be able to care for him at home again. I therefore allowed the hospital to put him into a nursing home when they discharged him. I did the appropriate research and found a home with a good reputation, one where a friend of mine worked. To my horror, when I visited him the first time, he was sitting in a wheelchair in the hallway with a puddle of urine underneath. The next time I visited, he was lying on his bed with only a sheet covering him. He kept saying to me, "They took my clothes. They took my clothes." He did not even have a Depends pad on! I immediately took steps to bring him back home.*

As she related this story, I realized that people with this type of neurological disease can't fend for themselves. In a busy, understaffed nursing home, they can easily become the most neglected patients. This could happen to Charles. He wouldn't be able to express his needs clearly—or even press a nurse call button. This conversation unequivocally convinced me that Charles would need to stay home.

I also spoke with another member of the Society for PSP whose husband had died. Her voice was so comforting, I just had to ask, "Did your husband go through a period of yelling constantly? If so, how did you handle it?"

She responded, "My husband didn't yell, but he threw things. I think it was because he was frustrated. I just continued to love him through this and accept him."

That advice hit me powerfully—and just at the right time. Charles's yelling had been going on for over a month, and I knew that it might continue for many more. Feeling exasperated, I wasn't sure I could continue to handle it. I don't know why the woman's simple sharing of being calm and gracious through such difficult episodes with her husband touched me so perfectly. But with her counsel, I committed myself to accepting the yelling—and Charles. Peace comforted me, instead of frustration overcoming me. How appropriate for the holiday season.

Caregiving Affirmation:
You'll be more at peace if you accept your loved one as is,
rather than futilely fighting the disease's symptoms.

SOMETHING WORSE THAN THE YELLING

But the yelling wasn't the worst of it.

Another personality change had been slowly occurring. I had noticed it over the previous year. Charles, in a very adorable way, began saying, even with his slurring speech, "I love you," to all of the female aides and nurses. When we went to his thirtieth high school reunion in Searcy, Arkansas, he told his former high school sweetheart that he loved her. When we returned home, he had his aide type a letter for him to send to her. In the letter, he talked about how he had always loved her. I knew that neurological diseases and their medications can cause inappropriate sexual feelings and an urge to express them. This had happened to the father of one of my brothers-in-law when the father developed Alzheimer's, so I didn't worry too much about these seemingly innocuous remarks.

Then Charles told me that he loved Deedee, his aide. This time it wasn't just a cute "I love you." He actually said that he was in love with her. I believed he truly felt that, but I tried to just chalk it up to the disease. But over time, it wore down my self-esteem, and my heart ached. When the caregiving became excruciating because of his yelling, I caught myself thinking, *Why are you still giving him this care? How can you keep doing this if he doesn't love you anymore?* I wished he had said "I love you" to *me* during this trying time. It hurt to not hear it at this point. Even though I know that he adored me throughout our marriage, it was still an effort to convince myself that this was just the disease.

I didn't realize, though, that Charles had started badgering Deedee. While his communication was limited, he had managed to make inappropriate sexual comments to Deedee. Deedee tried to handle this quietly on her own. But finally, she called me in tears one day and told me what Charles had been saying. "Oh my goodness, Deedee," I responded. "He told me that he loved you, but I didn't realize that he was harassing you!" While the yelling was starting to get better, now Charles's sexual comments pushed Deedee to nearly quitting again.

Now I'd finally put enough of the pieces together. Realizing the tremendous scope of Charles's problems with yelling and inappropriate sexual comments, I called Dr. Ravin. I needed her wisdom and concern. When she reached me later that night, she tenderly assured me that the yelling and inappropriate sexual thoughts were not Charles. She said, "Some people falsely think that when someone does these bad things, it is revealing the real person. That's just not so. This is not Charles. It is *not* who he really is. It is the disease."

Dr. Ravin's words helped Deedee cope, too. In addition, I worked with Dr. Ravin to increase the dose of the Seroquel, which began to work miraculously as the dose was titrated upward. Dr. Ravin also decreased the dose of the Parkinson's medication, Sinemet, which has been known to cause these types of behavioral and psychotic problems with prolonged use.

Slowly, peace began to return.

Caregiving Affirmation:
Remember that difficult personality changes are *not*
your loved one—they are the disease.

5

1999: Hanging On

TRANSITION TO HOME—CHARLES RETIRES

TRANSITION TO LIVING AT HOME

As of January 1, 1999, Charles would no longer be going in to his office at Web; he would no longer feel like part of the team, or contribute his expertise and passion to the work he loved. Instead of anticipating what many healthy retirees view as a positive life change, Charles had reluctantly slid downhill into retirement. The disease had conquered yet another part of Charles's life.

In late September of 1998, the founder of the company, Bob Fulton, had e-mailed Charles, reiterating what the two of them had talked about during a recent lunch date: "I expect that you have been giving some serious thought to retirement. It would be so good (right) for you to retire while you are still able to as your decision, not someone else's. . . . Seriously, Charles, I would encourage you to take this step as your own choice rather than have someone make it for you."

"Janet, do you think I should retire?" Charles asked, after showing me the e-mail.

"It's up to you, Charles," I responded, trying not to influence his decision but knowing that he couldn't physically handle going to work much longer.

Sadly, he agreed: "I probably should."

Later that fall, we got out his laptop computer and typed a list of the things he wanted to do when he retired. We also jotted down one way Web Industries might help—by allowing him to keep his computer and e-mail address, in order to stay in contact with the people there who meant so much to him. They agreed, and Charles dictated a letter that was e-mailed to Web employees:

> *I have an illness that's affecting my health; therefore, I intend to retire. This illness is a fatal disease that makes it difficult for me to contribute as best I can to Web Industries. Although many things are difficult for me now, I would like to make the contributions to Web that are still possible.*
>
> *These are some of the contributions I would like to carry over into my retirement. Delivering doughnuts and talking to the people at Framingham is something I would continue to enjoy. Since I plan on keeping up with my reading (or rather, having books read to me), I'll be collecting quotes to send out for the thought for the day. Also, anyone is welcome to respond and/or talk to me via e-mail. I would like to maintain regular calls to key people to encourage and support them. I hope to continue to support the work in Hungary. I would also like to remain working with the ESOP Association.*
>
> *On a more personal note, I plan to finish my book,* Paradoxes of Leadership, *and start a new book. I also want to keep in close contact with my family. A new project I'm planning is to write to and start helping to support people with PSP.*
>
> *All of you know how much of a workaholic I am, and so I want to start my education on how to relax and have fun. I welcome all of your phone calls and visits, and want to continue to build on the wonderful relationships created at Web.*

Just after the first of the year, Web moved Charles's computer, along with a combination printer and fax machine, into the study of our home.

RETIREMENT PARTY

Charles sat there for over two hours in the hotel ballroom with his body folded stiffly into a wingback chair. A pillow supported his hyperextended neck, another cushioned his puffy, cocked left arm, and a third raised his feet off the ground. Except for eating, his occasional glances to the right or left were the only movements he made all night. I'm doubtful, though, that he could see (due to his lack of peripheral vision and ability to intentionally move his eyes) the more than a hundred people sitting at the round tables in front of him—all of whom had come to honor him.

All night, I was afraid that Charles would start yelling at some point. I don't know if I thought about bringing the grapes or if I was just lucky enough to have them there. But whenever Charles appeared to become slightly agitated, I stuffed a grape in his mouth. He'd quietly chew and swallow. Then just like a baby bird waiting for the mother to place another worm in its mouth, Charles opened his mouth, awaiting the next grape. When he wasn't eating a grape, his mouth hung limply open until he'd give an occasional laugh or smile, showing that he just might be understanding what was going on around him.

Because it was already three months after his last day of work, the event was more of a tribute than a retirement party. The friends in attendance couldn't make the normal retirement wishes—to go have fun without the burden of work responsibilities. They all knew. They could clearly see that Charles's retirement wouldn't be blissful or carefree. But they had lots to say about his contribution to Web and, more especially, to their lives. A dozen people from various aspects of Charles's work and professional life gave moving accolades.

- John: "Charles knows how to acknowledge people."
- Vickie: "You gave us an opportunity to grow."
- Dick: "He always gave credit to others."
- Josh: "Charles wasn't a spectator in life. He participated in the fullest way."
- Charlie: "Charles had a burning passion for nurturing the human side in all of us."
- Donnie, the company president: "While Charles had a

marvelous intellect, his ego was way down there—you couldn't find it." He spoke tenderly about how hard it was to watch his friend slip away.

- Dan, one of Charles's best friends: "He gave grace to people at every walk and level."

- Bob, the company founder: "Charles is a rare person." To illustrate, he used the words *compassion, caring, under-standing, listening,* and *loving.*

Charlie, the sales manager whom Charles promoted out of operations years ago, created a funny and yet moving video. The title screen appeared: "*A Tribute to Charles,* starring Charles Edmunson." Then the screen flashed a warning: "The images of Charles in all shapes and sizes may not be suitable for younger viewers. Parental discretion is advised." Everyone laughed, remembering Charles in his "Charlie Buddha" stage, with his round belly and puffy, cheery cheeks, and then sleek and trim after his angioplasty.

The video showed many still pictures and action video of Charles with various Web employees over his twenty years at the company. At one point, Charlie used a clip from an in-house Web video made years ago in which Charles said, "Our manufacturing services are used in products that touch people's lives every day." Charlie aptly turned the words around to say, "Charles is a man that strived to touch people's lives every day." He finished the video with an illustration of a pumping heart and said, "You can't find a man with a bigger heart. Thank you, Charles. We love you."

Caregiving Affirmation:
Provide opportunities for your loved one to hear accolades.

After the presentations and video, we invited everyone to greet Charles while I took pictures of each one with him. Some hugged him; others kissed him on the forehead or touched his hair. Some just stood next to him. While some comfortably showed their affection, others awkwardly tried to carry on the necessarily one-way conversation. However each person interacted with Charles, compassion for him and awe at his life's work overflowed throughout the evening. What a bittersweet launch for Charles's transition to living at home.

CHARLES'S CONDITION WORSENS

ANOTHER HOSPITALIZATION

Ken, Charles's brother, had just visited. The first day Ken arrived, he spent most of the time in the bathroom, fighting a stomach virus he'd caught from his two-year-old daughter. After about twenty-four hours, though, he started to feel better, and we had a nice visit.

But the evening after Ken left, Charles started shaking all over, sweating profusely, and breathing with short, fast, shallow breaths. It scared me. I hadn't seen these symptoms before. Could they have been the result of being exposed to the virus Ken had? Or was he having a heart attack? Or was it a strange new aspect of this neurological disease?

What should I do? Charles couldn't talk well enough to tell me what he was feeling. I would have to make the decision.

When the sweating, shaking, and rapid breathing didn't subside, I loaded Charles into the car and we headed for the local hospital. Because of his past heart condition, they took him in right away and hooked him up to an electrocardiogram machine.

To my disappointment, the emergency room doctor insisted that Charles needed to be admitted for the night so that he could undergo the full round of cardiac enzyme tests, which could confirm or rule out a heart attack. He gave us the option to stay there in Framingham or to transport Charles to the larger hospital system at UMass Memorial Medical Center in Worcester.

At least that was an easy decision—UMass Memorial Medical Center was where Charles's doctors practiced. Emergency medical technicians wheeled him into an ambulance, and I followed the twenty miles down Route 9 to UMass Memorial Medical Center's emergency room, frightened.

They immediately took Charles to an area in the emergency room that wasn't really a room at all—just a space with a bed, surrounded by sliding curtains. They hooked him up to new machines; soon, we knew that his electrocardiogram, blood pressure, and temperature were all normal. As he lay there, he sweated profusely, absolutely drenching his shirt, and he continued to shake and gasp. The hospital staff members struggled to give Charles the attention that I felt he needed due to other competing emergencies. But upon my request, one of the nurses gave me some cold cloths. I stood beside Charles, periodically whispering calmly to him, "You'll be okay," and wiped his body continually for the next hour or so in an attempt to cool him.

As with previous emergency room experiences, it seemed like an eternity between visits by a nurse or doctor, because there was so much activity all around us. After I told and retold Charles's complicated story, staff members confirmed that they were simply waiting for a bed in the hospital to open up so they could officially admit him.

IT ALWAYS GETS MORE COMPLICATED

As midnight approached, I gave in to sheer exhaustion, slumping over the back of my stiff plastic chair and trying to rest. With my eyes closed, the sounds of the emergency room swam around in my dull consciousness—nurses coming and going, picking up drugs from the pneumatic tube system in front of us, attending to the patients to Charles's right and left. The older women to our right complained about a flare-up of some sort of digestive problem.

Then I overheard a discussion to our left between the doctor and a young woman. She described seeing bugs all over the doctor, the walls, and the ceiling. I figured that she was high on illicit drugs.

While fading in and out of a very light sleep, I thought I heard something move close to me. I opened my heavy eyes and saw a young woman with messy long blonde hair and wearing a flannel shirt and jeans standing right next to me—the one who'd been seeing bugs. She looked as if she was getting ready to pick up my purse.

I instinctively grabbed my purse and spoke firmly, asking her what she was doing and demanding that she go back to her bed. She obeyed and retreated behind the flimsy curtain. As I closed my eyes to rest again, I began to think that maybe she hadn't been getting ready to pick up my purse—maybe she already had picked it up and had been putting it back down. In a panic, I checked my purse and found all the cash missing. I jumped up to get the attention of the nearest nurse. She called the hospital campus police while keeping an eye on the blonde woman. As I further inspected my purse, I noticed that my credit cards and driver's license were also missing.

The young women denied taking anything when the police lieutenant questioned her. He had his assistant search her coat pockets, where my credit cards and license were hiding. Because I had been to the cash machine earlier that day, I knew I had at least three hundred dollars in my wallet, which the blonde woman must have taken. But the police couldn't find it. They instructed me to write a report of what had happened while they took her to the police station.

The next day, with Charles comfortably settled in a hospital room, the lieutenant returned to say the police had finally found the cash. The young woman had hidden about two hundred dollars in her coat and clothes; the rest, he shyly admitted, she had stuffed in her internal "crevices." He assured me that I could get it all back in a few days after the police used it for testimony against her in court.

Before Charles was discharged from the hospital, I picked up the money—some in a sealed plastic bag. I eventually took it to a bank, explaining my story to the wide-eyed teller. She took my word for the amount of money in the bag and gave me crisp new bills.

Some Positive Outcomes

Throughout this disease, some new insights would occasionally come to me. I wondered why they hadn't come sooner.

I typically can find creative solutions to problems. I did this many times in caring for Charles. But sometimes even the most obvious options didn't occur to me—sometimes someone else had to describe them, or I had to see them in action. Thankfully, I saw a wonderful solution in action during that hospital stay.

In cases of likely incontinence, the hospital used an extra cloth pad underneath the patient. We used these at home. But in addition to a Depends pad, the hospital used the cloth pads as the sole protection for the mattress overnight. They didn't use a condom catheter.

Though the Depends pads didn't catch all of the overnight urine, the pad underneath did.

I didn't think that using Depends pads overnight would work at home—and I thought that they might irritate Charles's skin and cause sores. But in the hospital, using special powder, he had no irritation or sores. Hooray! I now had an alternative to the dreaded condom catheter.

The catheter had negatively affected our relationship. Nothing else that I had to do for him produced more anger toward me than putting on a condom catheter each night. I was the bad guy. He kept asking me why I made him wear them—they were uncomfortable, and sometimes even painful. I hadn't known that another option existed; now, with this new easy solution, I wouldn't need to fight Charles each night to put on the catheter that he absolutely despised. No more hateful stares as I awkwardly positioned it just before bedtime. No more screams as I would inevitably catch pubic hairs in it as I took it off each morning. And no more frustration when it would occasionally pop off at night and urine would leak through all the bedsheets. Getting ready for bed at night finally became more peaceful. I wish I had known about this solution earlier, and that I had never used the condom catheter on Charles.

I also learned that hospitalizations are a reliable way to get a health insurance company to pay for new services. After Charles's few hospital experiences, the doctors ordered home visits by physical therapists and occupational therapists. These professionals helped me learn how to move Charles from car, to bed, and to toilet, as well as how to pick him up if he landed on the floor—all without straining my back.

GETTING DISCHARGED

Just as with the last hospital visit, Charles's symptoms improved within the first twenty-four hours. That made me certain that his problems developed from the virus Ken had shared when visiting—not a heart attack. This being a hospital, though, tests must be done! But with my pleading, this time the doctors discharged Charles after only two grueling nights.

What trauma to be dealing with Charles's mysterious shaking and sweating and then the theft of my money! Coping with a degenerative disease is overwhelming and relentless. And it always seemed during Charles's illness that at my time of greatest vulnerability, something else would always strike to test my strength. I accepted that it wasn't fair, but my acceptance still didn't make things any easier.

Caregiving Affirmation:
Give yourself credit for staying strong despite
being pushed to your limits.

The End of His "Daily Personal Victory"

For the last 1,675 days in a row, Charles had been faithful to the commitment he had made to himself in 1994—before the disease had shown its first insidious symptom—to run every day as his daily personal victory.

His determination when making that commitment resonated now in my mind because these latest experiences had traumatized and weakened him just enough to convince me that his running—and more recently, his walking—streak must end. I could no longer handle him by myself. I had to be the one to break the commitment he'd faithfully kept for over four years.

I couldn't come up with the words to tell Charles that it was finally time to stop, so I didn't say anything to him directly. We just no longer included a walk in our daily routine. Would he even notice that we weren't going anymore? I hoped not. But as heartbreaking as it was to end the routine, I found myself relieved of what had become an overwhelming and scary burden.

"No More Hospitals!"

That hospital stay convinced me that it would be our last. I vowed, "No more hospitals!" I didn't fully understand what this would mean. But I did know that nothing that the hospital offered would improve Charles's quality of life. In fact, these experiences tortured him.

A few months earlier, the nurse from Deedee's agency had visited. While sitting at our kitchen table, she asked, "Janet, have you considered signing a DNR for Charles?" I had never heard of a DNR. She went on to explain, "It stands for 'do not resuscitate.' It allows you and Charles to decide what measures you want taken in a medical emergency. And it provides a way for you to say that you just want comfort, or palliative, care—like pain control and oxygen."

Now after three horrible hospital stays within three months, I remembered that conversation and called Charles's primary care doctor. He explained that a DNR would allow us to determine ahead what type of treatments, or lack of treatments, we would want, such as feeding tubes and cardiopulmonary resuscitation (CPR). He agreed that the time was right to complete a DNR, so he sent me the paperwork. Once Dr. Ravin, Charles's primary neurologist, and I signed the DNR form, it was official. No extraordinary measures would be taken just to keep Charles alive should something happen. As instructed, I taped it in a prominent place—on the full-length mirror next to our bed.

Now What Have I Done?

With the DNR signed and posted, I had to explain the new procedures to all the caregivers. Darry had the hardest time understanding why I had done this. I could see the question, and almost disagreement, on his face. From his standpoint as Charles's aide, he needed to have a plan if Charles faced a medical emergency. "Shouldn't I call 911 for an ambulance?" he asked. This all went completely against Darry's instincts. It made him feel vulnerable and at risk in the responsibility he took so seriously.

I replied, "No, don't call 911 under any circumstances. If something happens, call my pager."

And then the reality hit.

What would I actually do if Darry called saying that Charles was choking or looked like he was having a heart attack or some other emergency? I knew for certain that Charles did not need another grueling hospital visit. But what would I do? What had I done in signing the DNR? Like Darry, I felt completely defenseless.

Would Charles Approve?

I knew deep in my heart that the DNR decision was right for

me and Charles. But people would always ask, when they learned about the DNR, if this was Charles's wish and if I had talked this over with him.

I hadn't—not because I didn't want to, but because I'd found I just couldn't address this issue with him. While Charles could still communicate, he didn't want to believe he was dying. I felt that if I brought up this discussion, he would resist even talking about it. And there was more. When he was frustrated, he would sometimes shout at me, "You are going to be glad when I die!" And as he experienced greater and greater losses, he would more frequently yell, "I wish I were dead!" He felt despair that he could no longer do things for himself, so he couldn't believe that I could stand it. I felt that talking about a DNR, as well as the health care proxy we needed to sign, would make him feel as if I actually *would* be glad when he died—and the quicker, the better. But that wasn't my motivation.

At that point in the disease, Charles couldn't talk well enough to have this discussion. But I felt that if he could have communicated his desires, he would have agreed to the DNR. His life had been about making a difference in the world. Merely subsisting through means of a feeding tube or other heroic measures, rather than truly living, wouldn't have fit with the mission he'd recited and lived each day.

Caregiving Affirmation:
Focus on the quality, not the length, of your loved one's life.

JUST WHEN I NEEDED IT

That last hospital encounter must have triggered something at Blue Cross Blue Shield of Massachusetts. Mary, one of the case managers, called me at work. Her caring and supportive tone alleviated my initial fears that Blue Cross might deny care. And her assistance helped lead me through some important decisions.

I felt comfortable explaining to Mary the struggles I'd had with Charles—the yelling, the physical losses, and signing the DNR. During one of our conversations, she asked if I had considered hospice. I'd decided long ago that I would take advantage of hospice, but I didn't know when it would be time to do so. When would I know that Charles was within six months of dying—the standard point at which hospice takes over a person's care?

MY EARLIER HOSPICE EXPERIENCE

My family had experienced the tender care of hospice when my father died in 1995. Dad smoked and drank heavily most of his life. He admitted that these lifestyle choices would one day kill him—and they did.

After two operations—one to remove his larynx and add a voice box, and the other to take out additional cancer—as well as chemotherapy and radiation, his health faded over two years. His cancer had spread to his lungs.

Although Dad appeared reasonably healthy until the weekend he died, I'm sure his pain was worse than he let on. Had we known how close to death he really was, Mom would have enlisted the aid of hospice sooner.

The weekend that Dad died, he must have finally given up. He quickly went into a semicoma, which triggered Mom's call to hospice. She also called my four sisters and brother, who quickly caught flights to Florida. However, Charles and I were visiting a friend in Philadelphia for the weekend. I hadn't left a phone number with anyone, because I hadn't expected Dad's quick decline. Fortunately, I decided to call Mom on Saturday morning from Philadelphia just to check on him. I left Philadelphia immediately, worrying that I would miss the opportunity to tell him good-bye, and that I loved him. The hospice nurse thought Dad could die at any time.

When I arrived, he was still alive, though very much in a coma. All of my siblings were already there. He seemed unaware of me, his gaunt face unshaven and his mouth hanging open. The hospice nurse, sitting in the corner of the room, greeted me and calmly explained the dying process—what was probably, for her, the sixth time. The particular hospice that Mom used provided nursing care around the clock for Dad, something that that program regularly did during what was expected to be the last three days of life. The nurse administered regular doses of morphine, swabbed Dad's mouth, and provided all the other hygienic care he needed.

As night approached, Dad was still hanging on. We took two-hour shifts in pairs to stay with him throughout the night. We read passages to him from the Bible, sang songs from the hymnals Mom had, and just stayed close and held his cold hands.

When the hospice nurse saw signs of Dad's impending death, everyone was awakened, and we all gathered around him, holding each other's hands and sharing our love. In the very early morning, on Halloween, Dad finally died peacefully, without pain and surrounded by his family. The home environment allowed us to experience Dad's last breath in the quiet of his own bedroom—with no one to bother us, no one to ask permission, and no sterile hospital rooms. And we all felt richer and closer for the experience.

RELIEF AT LAST

I began to believe that Charles wouldn't last the year. His physical losses had mounted even more quickly than expected, and his health had declined sharply. He didn't seem cognizant much of the time, he couldn't talk, and he couldn't do anything for himself.

At my call, hospice representatives came immediately and evaluated Charles's condition. They called Dr. Ravin, who agreed that Charles likely had less than six months to live and would be a good candidate for hospice.

But then I worried. What if Charles lived longer than six months? Would I have to withdraw Charles from hospice, just when his condition would probably be worsening? Would we have used up all of our allotted hospice services before we really needed them? Was now the right time to do this?

Then the panic hit hard—I had signed the DNR. How would I know what to do without hospice?

Again Mary, the insurance case manager, assured me and encouraged me not to worry. "We'll figure it out as we go," she said. I am indebted to Mary for mentioning hospice to me at that time. Without her suggestion, I'm sure I would have waited quite some time before looking into hospice.

I officially enrolled Charles in hospice in February 1999, and he

lived a little over a year longer. I worried every six months when Blue
Cross reviewed his case, but thankfully, the company continued to
allow his hospice care.

My New Safety Net

Hospice became my safety net. I can still remember my
immense relief at knowing that I was no longer alone. I had someone to help me coordinate Charles's care. What peace to know that
if he had an emergency, hospice would be there.

The philosophy of hospice is to provide *comfort care*, not to use
heroic measures. The phrase comfort care might at first seem quite
passive. But in my experience, they represented a proactive
approach. The hospice workers did whatever it took to keep
Charles comfortable during his natural death; he didn't have a
stressful hospital death. I found consolation in knowing that the
drugs, such as morphine, that he might need were already approved
and in the refrigerator.

Now I had a plan. If something happened to Charles, I would
call hospice.

Caregiving Affirmation:
Consider hospice sooner versus later;
the support will bring you relief.

Caregiving Essentials

The hospice-style makeover of our home began when a delivery
man wheeled in a cold, chrome hospital bed, loaded with gadgets to
lift Charles up, down, forward, and backward, and placed it in the
same spot where our warm cherrywood queen-size four-poster had
been. A white hospital blanket replaced the soft mauve, sage green,
and mellow gold flowered comforter that had matched the wallpaper
border in the room. The soothing watercolor picture of the Chain
Bridge in Budapest still looked down on the bed area, so at least we
still had a reminder of the time we'd spent walking hand in hand
across that romantic nineteenth-century bridge, a string of lights glit-
tering along each side. Hanging on the wall opposite the new bed,

our plaster of Paris angel mask could continue her watch over us. Charles had presented the angel to me as a gift many years earlier when we were decorating our first home in Atlanta. He thought the angel, with its small face, blonde hair, and blue eyes, resembled me.

The rolling table that accompanied the hospital bed neatly kept handy many of the supplies now needed for Charles's care—moisture barrier, plastic pail for washing, disposable gloves, and hairbrush. Beside it stood a Diaper Genie, in which the aides and I placed the soiled Depends pads. This disease had brought Charles's body back to infancy.

Charles's burgundy lifter recliner found a new home in our bedroom because it was a comfortable alternative to the bed and the wheelchair, the only places in which he now spent his entire day. And the innovative contraption helped ease the difficulty of moving Charles in and out of the recliner by actually lifting up the back of the entire chair. But that meant the fold-up treadmill—the one given to him by friends in 1996—had to move down the hall to the study. He'd tried to use it on days with inclement weather. Helping him onto the treadmill, I would hold his arm as we slowly increased the speed from a slow walk to a faster one. Eventually, knowing that the rubber belt was not under his control scared him too much; he would panic and lose his footing. I rushed to stop the treadmill before he fell. After a number of attempts over a few weeks failed, I folded it up and put it in a corner.

For the last few months, though, I had been regularly using the treadmill. I preferred to walk and run outside, but using the treadmill at least gave me the opportunity to exercise and stay with Charles in the morning before the aide arrived. And when I started to get bored with pounding my feet on the moving belt, I could glance up to see the watercolor picture featuring the TGI Friday's restaurant on Exeter Street in Boston's Back Bay. Charles and I had frequented that restaurant when we were dating, and we'd shared an Oreo cookie ice cream drink there at about 1:30 AM the first day of our honeymoon. We'd carried that watercolor with us to all of the houses we'd owned.

I don't know how Charles felt about these new practical caregiving essentials occupying our once private space. But the presence of these inanimate intruders assured me that we would now be supported by hospice. And that knowledge, along with the memories triggered by our pictures and the angel, gave me comfort and peace.

More Than I Expected

I got more than I could have dreamed of with hospice.

Dianne, the primary nurse assigned to Charles, visited only twice a week, but her interventions with Dr. Ravin helped stop the yelling, kept his bowels moving, got his medications modified as needed, and improved the care and hygiene the aides and I provided him, and, most importantly, gave me someone to call with absolutely any question or concern I had. With Dianne working on our behalf, we no longer needed to see any of Charles's doctors. That meant that I didn't need to take the time off work to take Charles, and he didn't need to go through the ordeal of traveling there. And Dianne or one of the hospice on-call nurses was available day and night.

Dianne skillfully came up with a solution to almost every critical problem I brought to her. Sometimes the solution didn't work, but then she'd tenaciously try another one. Her expertise helped us prevent many of the terrible problems people confined to home typically encounter. For instance, one of the first practices she instituted was the use of a petroleum jelly moisture barrier all around Charles's groin and buttocks before putting on a new Depends pad. The aides and I had been using one of the brand-name powders, but we soon found the petroleum jelly product provided better protection against chapping.

Besides Dianne, we also had other kinds of health care practitioners as needed. In the beginning, hospice sent an occupational therapist to the house. She helped us modify how we moved Charles into difficult places—such as out of bed and into the shower. And she made recommendations for modifications around the house to ease our difficulties.

Hospice focused not only on the patient but also on the caregiver. The social worker they assigned worked with both Charles and me. Of course, the social worker struggled in helping Charles, as he could no longer talk clearly enough to be understood, so we eventually ended those sessions. But the social worker helped me feel comfortable in the way I was handling the caregiving process. These sessions forced me to slow my hectic pace and focus on my emotional needs. She made me feel sane throughout this insane experience.

Hospice also provided a spiritual advisor for Charles. David, who also served as a pastor of a local church, visited Charles nearly every week. Charles continued to have deep religious questions, so I'm sure that David's sharing of spiritual thoughts comforted him. The social worker remarked that Charles would often be somewhat agitated when she was with him, but then when David came, he immediately calmed down and became attentive. David seemed to help Charles think through his struggles with faith, meeting a need that I couldn't.

Hospice had a network of trained volunteers that filled other needs we had. Though they couldn't serve as aides, they could be with Charles for an hour or two when we had a gap in the aides' schedule. In addition to the volunteers, hospice also connected us with a local church, St. Ann's, on the holidays.

At Easter, a kind couple with a shy daughter about ten years old came to our door, dressed in their nice Easter outfits. They were carrying two large shopping bags filled with everything from soup to dessert, as well as beverages and a flower for the table. I introduced them to Charles. Even though the young girl seemed somewhat afraid, I thought it was wonderful that she was being given the chance to experience volunteerism at such an early age. And what a treat the food was for Charles and me, especially because I had never been much of a cook. We experienced this same gratitude at Thanksgiving that year, too.

Hospice and Blue Cross expanded our coverage of home health aides. With the additional resources, hospice took on the role of working with the agencies to find the aides we needed—a very difficult task because aides were in very short supply. But the headache was predominantly on hospice's shoulders now, not mine.

My fright after signing the DNR quickly vanished with hospice on my side.

CHARLES'S DAY AT HOME

After awakening at 5:30 AM each weekday, I had time to walk or jog on the treadmill and get my shower before the morning aide arrived. Meanwhile, Charles coasted awake with the local news on the television after I had inserted a torpedo-shaped suppository to help encourage a bowel movement—which often wouldn't come.

Carlos, the short, stocky Brazilian aide, arrived at 6:30. For the first task of the day, he took Charles through his stretching routine. Unfortunately, no matter how much I tried to demonstrate and explain, Carlos never caught on to how slowly these exercises should be conducted. I'd hear Charles yelp in pain when his rigid muscles reached the end of their resistance. I struggled with what to do: Should I have stopped Carlos from doing these altogether? Should I have been the one to do them for Charles instead? My indecision meant I had to tolerate Charles's discomfort, and I hoped he could tolerate it, too. His muscles needed the movement so that they wouldn't atrophy and stiffen, causing him more pain.

Hospice replaced our original shower chair with an elongated one that extended to just outside of the shower. After maneuvering the wheelchair into place, Carlos lifted Charles onto the end of the chair, swiveled his legs inside the stall, and then lifted him again to scoot him into the center of the chair. He leaned Charles toward the side wall to help keep him from falling over. Carlos and other aides found Charles's buttocks to be the hardest part to wash. In the past, Charles had been able to stand and hold on to the bar at the front of the shower, once lifted to his feet. Now we couldn't trust that anymore. Imagine the difficulty of trying to wash a person at the same time you are trying to keep him from falling.

Sharing the bathroom (I'd resigned myself to this unavoidable lack of privacy), I continued to put on my makeup and blow-dry my hair, making small talk while Carlos proceeded to brush Charles's teeth with the electric toothbrush. Earlier in the year, Carlos had had Charles swish clean water and spit into a plastic cup to rinse. But now it seemed like Charles had forgotten how to spit. He just swallowed the toothpaste mixed with saliva. We switched to natural toothpaste without fluoride to make this new routine a little safer.

Having put out Charles's and my clothes the night before, I dressed in the powder room in the front hall. Meanwhile, Carlos placed Charles back on the bed and first put the Depends pads on, with two extra Dignity pads. To make dressing Charles easier, we'd found a style of cotton pants from JCPenney with an elastic waistband, eliminating the struggle with the tight fit, zipper, and belt of other pants. Wearing one of his attractive golf shirts, Charles looked presentable for his long day at home.

As I prepared to walk out the door to head to work, Carlos wheeled Charles into the kitchen and fed him dry cereal from a cup. Carlos held the cup and lifted it up to Charles's mouth, because Charles could no longer coordinate such movements. Carlos also gave him his pills mixed into a small bowlful of applesauce. He had lost his ability to swallow pills whole and now instinctively chewed them all. I eliminated a few supplementary pills from the regimen, such as odd vitamins, coenzyme Q10, and ginkgo biloba, to make this task easier, and a little tastier.

Unfortunately, while Charles could still chew and swallow his food and pills, liquids began to cause him to cough and choke. So Carlos mixed a spoonful or two of a powdery substance called Thick-It into the orange juice and other drinks to change their consistency, allowing for safer swallowing. I took a sip once of Thick-It in cranberry juice, wondering if it made the drinks taste bad, and thankfully found that it didn't.

On most mornings, Deedee arrived at the house at 8:30 to assume the aide responsibilities for the day. Now at home instead of at Charles's office, she got into a new routine—*Live with Regis and Kathy Lee* and reruns of *Little House on the Prairie* on the TV while Charles took his morning nap, reading books to Charles, and, even more frequently, having him listen to tapes during the afternoons. The days went better for her now that Charles was more peaceful due to the right balance of medications.

Deedee continued producing the "thought for the day" on his behalf, getting new thoughts from the leadership books she read to Charles. But now, instead of responding with the words "Thought

for the day" when he heard a concept he agreed with, he could only
say, "Wow!" But she knew what he meant. Later in the year, though,
he lost the ability to say even that, and Deedee could no longer continue sending the e-mailed thoughts. We changed the schedule to
one thought a week and I took over the task, looking for a quote
from Charles's newly published book, *Paradoxes of Leadership.* I didn't
want him to lose this form of communication. The regular e-mail
prompted his friends and colleagues to send messages back, which
lifted his spirits.

Charles could no longer hold on to the toilet's handrails, so all his
bowel movements had to happen while he was in bed with his
Depend's pad on. By mid-afternoon, Charles became uncomfortable
moving his bowels. Not able to talk and tell us what was wrong, he
would grunt loudly to get Deedee's attention. She'd turn him to his
right side, then his left. She tried a heating pad on his stomach. For
months, nothing seemed to work. Finally, with the persistent help of
our hospice nurse, we found the right regimen of heavy-duty laxa-
tives for him to drink and take in suppository form. I would cheer
out loud when a bowel movement finally came, dumping into his
Depend's pad, because he would then be out of his daily pain.
Cleaning up the movement was not nearly as difficult as making it
through his two-hour agony every afternoon.

At the request of the hospice nurse, I kept a notebook for recording any progression of symptoms or difficulties that happened during
the day. At the end of her shift, Deedee jotted down significant
issues, such as when Charles was uncomfortable and the size of the
bowel movement, if any. The notebook also became a great way for
me to communicate with the aides about anything special that might
be needed for the next day. I carried a pager (cell phones weren't yet
commonplace) in case the aides couldn't reach me on my work
phone. It rarely beeped, but I felt more comfortable knowing that
they could reach me anytime.

Charles started complaining about "gucky hands"—another new
quirk caused by the degeneration taking place in his brain. I guess
his brain pumped out mixed-up messages, giving him these odd sen-
sations. Working with Dianne, we increased the dosage of the mira-

cle drug Seroquel that alleviated the yelling, and soon the "gucky hand" feeling went away.

A team of hospice volunteers filled the one-hour gap between the time Deedee left and Darry, the evening aide, arrived. Our neighbors' teenage son also covered a few days, and I paid him an hourly wage. This pattern allowed me to work a full day.

The volunteers soon started filling a friendship role for Charles— and they did so masterfully. They read aloud to Charles the wonderful tributes people had written. Or they brought other books and articles to read. Some even sang songs or played music they thought would be special to him. One day I noticed a Livingston Taylor CD in the stack. (He's the brother of singer James Taylor.) I thought it was odd that a volunteer played Charles these songs, because most aides would typically play soothing classical music. Then I learned that Maggie, the bubbly volunteer with long blonde hair, was Livingston Taylor's wife.

At about 5:30 PM, Darry's routine started. He took Charles for a walk outside in his wheelchair and then repeated the morning stretches and gave him a quick shower. Charles continued to sweat profusely during the day, so I'm sure he enjoyed this end-of-day cleanup.

Because we no longer put Charles in the car for outings, I bought his frozen yogurt on my way home from work. Every night, I stopped at the Framingham rest stop on the Massachusetts Turnpike, which was only a few miles from home. The cashiers at the TCBY frozen yogurt counter soon started recognizing me and remembering my regular order. In addition to Charles's frozen yogurt cone, I bought myself a small chocolate cone that I devoured on the way home. Once in the car, I put Charles's cone in the tall plastic drinking glass I kept in the car's cup holder, picking it up only periodically to lick the drips. At home, I quickly placed it in an opening of the plastic webbed basket in the freezer that provided safe storage until he was ready for it after dinner. I enjoyed providing this delicious pleasure for him.

After I had changed from my work clothes into comfortable jeans or a sweat suit, Darry would leave Charles and me alone to give me time to talk to Charles. Touching his shoulder or stroking his hair, I

shared with him my ups and downs of the day while his engaging
brown eyes stared into mine. I couldn't be sure if he understood
what I was saying, but I talked as if he did. I still wanted him to feel
a part of my life.

To encourage him, I read special e-mails that he received and
talked to him about responses people had sent regarding his book.
I hoped that these would pick up his spirits and allow him to realize that he was still having an influence, even though he could no
longer write or carry on a conversation. The only reply he could
make was to look longingly into my eyes. I ended my conversation
with "I love you."

Then I headed to the kitchen to make our meager dinner—pasta
and sauce with frozen vegetables thrown in or heated-up frozen dinners—unless it was a Tuesday or Friday, when either Cal or Deedee
made us dinner. During our meal, I mostly talked directly to Darry,
with Charles just listening in and rarely giving any indication that he
was following along.

After his cherished frozen yogurt, Charles chewed his evening
pills mixed with chocolate pudding. I'm sure the green food supplements and other pills didn't taste good even with the chocolate, but
Charles didn't react visibly to them.

Then Darry prepared Charles for bed—brushing his teeth, transferring him into the bed, changing his Depends and Dignity pads,
and rolling him to his left side for sleep.

Charles now enjoyed the best sleep he'd had since before the
symptoms of his disease began to appear. The neurologist prescribed
Seconal, a barbiturate and thus a controlled substance—finally, a
solution that really worked. I got up only a couple of times in the
night when I went to the bathroom, and then I would roll him to
his other side.

Before I lay down, I put Franz Schubert's *Symphony No. 5 in B-
flat Major*, or other classical or New Age music, on the CD player to
create a peaceful environment for our sleep. Then I read *Man's Search
for Meaning* by Victor Frankl or *Men Are from Mars, Women Are from
Venus* by John Gray, relaxing into some of the most peaceful sleep
that I, too, had had in a long time.

FEELING RESPONSIBLE

Feeling completely responsible for Charles, I was almost ready to call his friends and make them feel guilty for not coming by—until I talked to Mike.

Mike was one of the hospice volunteers who spent an hour with Charles on various late afternoons between the morning and evening shifts of our aides. I usually didn't see him, as I was still at work. But I did notice his comforting smile and voice. One day I arrived home early when Mike was leaving. We chatted at the front door on his way out onto the porch. His words helped me through this anxious time.

Although some of Charles's colleagues—especially a few of his very closest friends—had visited him quite regularly throughout his illness and subsequent retirement, I had recently noticed that they weren't coming much at all anymore. My heart ached as I wondered whether Charles recognized their absence, and whether he felt lonely and abandoned.

To Charles, nothing was more important than relationships. During his first year of retirement, a number of friends had committed to seeing him often. Bob, his company's founder, came the most regularly and shared management books with Charles, as well as his humor and infectious laugh. Michelle from the Framingham plant also visited frequently, bringing along one of the other managers or workers with her. They talked about the politics at the plant, how various employees were doing, and the latest issues for the business. Charles's speech was slurred, but he said, "Wow!" quite clearly when someone said or read something profound, which reinforced the reward each felt in visiting. But as the disease progressed and Charles could no longer talk, his friends found it more difficult to visit. Even I found it hard to carry on a one-way conversation with him, so I could imagine how awkward his friends felt.

While Mike and I chatted, I thanked him for visiting and mentioned that the hospice volunteers now played an important role as friends for Charles. I told him that many of Charles's colleagues and friends had stopped coming by.

Mike's eyes tenderly focused on me and he said, "I understand." Then he revealed a personal story that helped me to understand, too. "I have a very good friend who has multiple sclerosis," he said, leaning on the frame of the open front door. "Prior to my friend's illness, we'd get together with three other buddies quite regularly, to play cards, talk, and enjoy each other. We were really close." Then Mike looked away, and his face revealed his guilty feelings. He said, "As time went on, my friend's MS progressed, keeping him in bed, unable to do much of anything. We all had a hard time talking to him and understanding him. Our two other close friends stopped visiting. I tried to keep going, but my visits got further and further apart. Now I can barely get myself to go once every five weeks or so; I find it too painful to see my friend so helpless."

But then he said, looking at me once again, his eyebrows furrowed as if a new truth was dawning on him, "While I have such a difficult time visiting my very closest friend with MS, I have no problem being with Charles in his condition. Maybe it's because I don't have that prior close relationship with him, like I have with my friend."

Now my eyes lit up with new awareness. "That explains why many of Charles's friends who were so good at visiting him earlier in the disease haven't come by recently," I remarked. I realized that Charles's friends had probably stopped visiting because it was too painful and difficult for them to see him deteriorating so much.

After Mike left, I decided not to make any more proactive phone calls to encourage visitors. Even though I was disappointed that Charles's friends didn't visit as much, I began to celebrate the strength of character of those who did visit and endure seeing Charles so helpless. I believe he rewarded their efforts with the sparkle and intensity of his eyes as he looked directly into theirs—his only way to communicate.

Caregiving Affirmation:
Expect that some people will find it too difficult to
visit your loved one. That's okay—it doesn't mean
that they've stopped caring.

LOST COMMUNICATION

"Talk to me about contemplating silence," Ted Koppel asked
Morrie Schwartz (profiled in *Tuesdays with Morrie*) in one of his
ABC News *Nightline* interviews. Morrie had amyotrophic lateral
sclerosis (also called Lou Gehrig's disease), which was slowly stealing
the volume of his voice. He replied that in thinking about the
inevitable loss of speech, he had reflected on the question "What will
it be like when I cannot articulate anything . . . or ask for something
. . . or say something that is in my heart . . . ?"

Then Ted mentioned that Morrie's best friend was losing his
hearing. "He, without hearing, and you, without speech, will be
sitting there together contemplating. What do you think that is
going to be like?" Ted asked. "There's going to be lots of love passing between us," Morrie replied.

Now Charles's speech had slipped away, like the sun setting—
slowly going away and then, before you knew it, gone. Initially, his
speech became slurred and garbled. Even Deedee, who spent the
most time with him, had trouble translating. The struggle to verbally
express his needs frustrated Charles to the point of anger, which
explained some of his yelling. But it also frustrated me and the others caring for him. As his ability to verbalize declined, I kept trying
to decipher what he was saying. Rarely, it seemed, did I get it right.
The discouraged look in his eyes told me that much. Parents must
experience this type of frustration when their toddlers mumble
words, thinking they are clearly communicating. The parents try this,
then that, interpreting what they think the child wants—and nothing
works. Finally the child breaks into an all-out wail. How frustrating to
not be able to figure out the needs and wants of their little loved one!
Distressed, I often had to work hard to convince myself that I was
doing the best I could.

Eventually, Charles was down to just an occasional "Wow." And
then just grunts and groans.

When Charles lost his speech, he lost much more. With other diseases, people who lose their ability to talk can at least make gestures to let others know their needs and wants. Because of Charles's apraxia, his brain couldn't direct his muscles to respond on command. Apraxia is a neurological disorder that keeps those who have it from being able to search their minds for the movements they want to make. Apraxia prohibited him from using nonverbal skills such as squeezing a hand once to mean yes and twice to mean no, or lifting one finger for yes and two fingers for no. All I and his aides could do was guess at his needs. I used my intuition and looked intensely into his eyes to determine if I had succeeded in solving his problem.

At the time, I didn't even try to put myself in Charles's place, because my feelings were plenty to deal with themselves. But as I reflect now, I still can't even imagine the intense frustration he must have felt but been unable to communicate. Eventually, he seemed to resign himself to his mute plight and gave up trying to express himself.

I asked the hospice nurse, Dianne, how I would know if he was in pain or uncomfortable. "Just look at his brow," she said. "If it furrows, chances are something is still not right." Her answer gave me confidence that I would be able to identify when he had a serious problem. But then I still had to resort to exasperating trial and error to determine what to do about it.

I also had to be mindful of how others talked around Charles. Often they seemed to forget he was there. I tried to turn things around and bring the questions and discussion back to Charles, wanting him to feel included. Most harmful, though, was when people talked about Charles in front of him.

Charles had always feared not being able to talk. He had been an articulate communicator, eloquent in his explanations and masterful at asking probing questions. Now, the deep conversations that were a hallmark of our relationship had completely evaporated. I now had the sole responsibility for our communication. I usually made simple comments or held short, one-way conversations. I very rarely went into a long soliloquy. I had never found it easy to just gab about things. I responded better once given an invitation via a thoughtful question. That was the way our conversations used to flow—I would pose an issue or problem, Charles would ask questions, I would respond. Now this limited communication proved tough and unfulfilling for me, and I'm sure it was the same for him, too. Had he recognized that I was talking to him less? All of my true conversations at home seemed to be confined to the aides or visitors, with Charles just listening in.

I began to wonder what Charles comprehended from the dialogue around him. Sometimes he appeared to be with us. Other times I sensed that he had given up. I'd get a clue from a laugh at just the right spot that he must actually be following along with the discussion. Then it would appear from his faraway look that he either didn't understand or couldn't follow what was being said. I was torn about this situation. On one hand, I hoped that he was aware of his surroundings and could understand the conversations, because he'd always loved lively discussion. But on the other hand, I hoped that he wasn't totally cognitive so that he couldn't understand that he was trapped in his body. Wouldn't that be too hard for him to bear if he was totally mindful of it?

As the year rolled on, Charles's smiles and laughter became less and less frequent, until both disappeared from his repertoire. He no longer showed any feelings. He seemed numb to daily existence, almost on autopilot. My heart ached at the loss of his engaging smile and jovial laugh. No longer talking, smiling, laughing, or showing emotion—was Charles the man I married? Was *he* still there?

Nonetheless, I believe, as Morrie said, that love still flowed between us.

Caregiving Affirmation:
Let the love flow, even when all else is lost.

THE CHALLENGE OF MANAGING AIDES

Whether I hired aides myself or an agency sent them, managing them could sometimes be a challenge. For most of our needs, we had great aides—Deedee, Darry, and Carlos—and they stayed with us for a number of years. Each of them had a unique and sometimes unconventional pattern with Charles, and they required relatively little oversight. However, other aides who cycled in and out were a different story.

I found it difficult to always give clear instructions. No matter how many lists I wrote and duties I described, I couldn't think of everything. Many of these transient aides only kept up with the minimum requirements. They would often leave dirty dishes in the sink. Urine stains and bowel movement accidents on the carpet were not appropriately cleaned up, and Charles's soiled clothes and bed linens wouldn't be washed. Because I tend to avoid confrontation, I struggled with finding a way to give the aides instructions without telling them how to do their job. I often was vague—or simply said nothing at all.

I noticed one day that one of the temporary aides fed Charles salad dressing from a small restaurant takeout container in the refrigerator. Had the aide thought that it was pudding? I struggled with whether to talk to him about this or just let it go. All I did was toss out four other containers of leftover takeout salad dressing so that it wouldn't happen again. But inside, I seethed.

I faced another challenge in coordinating between shifts of aides. Unfortunately, I initially didn't set up a fail-safe system to make sure that Charles wasn't left alone after the morning aide left. The morning aide had a tight time frame between the end of his shift with Charles and his next job, and just expected that Charles's aide for the next shift would eventually show up. So he left our house promptly by 8:30 AM, often before the next aide arrived. A few times, the second-shift aide didn't show up at all—either the aide called in sick and I didn't get notified, or something else thwarted the aide's arrival.

Imagine Charles lying in bed for hour after hour in the morning without anyone there, feeling abandoned and frightened. He couldn't do anything on his own. What must he have been thinking? Because at the time I was taking a train to work and leaving the house before the morning aide was finished, I didn't learn of any problems until sometime after I arrived at work. And the scary part was that a couple of times I learned that no one was with Charles only because I made a call home. What if I hadn't made that call? Charles would have been alone all day without anyone to feed him, change his

Depends pad, entertain him, or move him to protect his body from bedsores. I cringe to think of that possibility.

When I would discover such a problem, my hands and voice would shake as I rushed to call in some temporary help—a neighbor or a local friend—to get someone into the house until I could arrive home. Each of them described finding the same scene on their arrival at the house. "When I got in," one said, "Charles's clothes were drenched from his profuse sweating. His body was shaking and he was breathing heavily." How frightened he must have been, feeling utterly deserted. Until someone actually arrived in the house, we had no way to tell him that we knew about his plight—he couldn't answer the phone if we called.

After this happened a few times, I developed a prevention system with the morning aide. He was to call and leave me a message at work before he left the house on the days that the next aide did not arrive on time. This plan still had flaws, but at least it allowed me to find out immediately on arriving at work that there might be a problem. If I called home and the second-shift aide did not answer, I began my search to get someone into the house as quickly as possible.

Mondays continued to be a problem for me in finding aides. When I knew in advance that I would not have an aide, I would ask Gerard, Charles's former driver and early morning helper. His job was sometimes flexible enough to allow him to spend the day with Charles. But I really was stuck when the agency wouldn't tell me until Monday morning that they didn't have an aide for that day. That often left me taking a sick day off from work to care for Charles, exacerbating my already tremendous office workload.

But even when it looked like everything was all set, something invariably happened. For example, an agency we had just started to work with promised to send an aide one Monday, letting me know the aide's name. But the aide didn't show up. About an hour after his scheduled start time, I called, perturbed, and said, "The aide hasn't arrived. Is he lost, or is something wrong?" The agency director acted surprised and said, "I just talked to him. He should be there soon. He's on his way." But still no aide came. The next few times I called back, the director gave the same response—that the aide was on his way. The aide never did show, and the director never explained what really happened. When this event repeated itself the next week with the same agency director, I knew then that he'd never had an aide scheduled. I believe he lied to us. What a relief when another agency finally found Antonio to take on the Monday schedule. He connected with Charles immediately and became our stability on the day of the week that I'd come to dread.

But working with aides wasn't all hassles. I found that one of Charles's favorite sayings, "None of us is as smart as all of us," was true. Though I often got frustrated with the things aides wouldn't do correctly or carefully, I did find that they helped me discover solutions to quite a few caretaking problems.

For example, one day we had a new temporary aide who was a nursing student. She noticed that Charles's tongue was caked with black goo. As she cleaned it with a toothbrush, she found that it was layered about one eighth of an inch thick. How long had that crud been accumulating? Had Charles been able to taste any of his food with such a thick coating on his tongue? In discussions with the hospice nurse, we hypothesized that the sticky liquid lactulose, the powerful laxative that finally moved Charles's bowels, had probably initiated the problem.

Deedee always came up with great new suggestions. As Charles became totally dependent on us to roll him over from side to side, Deedee suggested we buy a satin sheet. It could be used as a draw sheet folded under the middle portion of his body to make sliding him from side to side easier.

Another struggle I faced was getting Charles's golf shirts off while he lay in bed. I fought with removing that last sleeve every time, his scrunched-up arm hitting his face. One day I observed Deedee doing it in such a simple and easy way. I put her technique into practice immediately. Even though it was only one small improvement in my care of Charles, it meant one less hassle.

When we started getting weekend aides through hospice, my life was simplified even more. The weekend aides came from a new agency that had a network of Ugandans as staff home health aides. Almost every one of them provided quality care, often surpassing my expectations. These aides became like family—relationships I would sorely miss after Charles died.

Now with Deedee, Darry, Carlos, Antonio, and the Ugandans, the difficulty of aide management decreased, taking an overwhelming pressure off me.

Caregiving Affirmation:
Plan to actively manage your aides—and learn from them, too.

I'VE ALREADY LOST HIM

A storm had been building over many months between two of my staff members at work. Finally, the storm hit. They blew up at each other. Although the conflict had been expected, I didn't feel it was necessary. When each person would talk to me individually, it appeared to me that they both had off-kilter perceptions of the other's intentions. But I wasn't effective in helping them see each other clearly.

I needed Charles's help. Problems like that one were just the sort that he and I would discuss together when he was well. Back then, we'd go for a walk, hand in hand, down Commonwealth Avenue in Newton. I'd bring up my latest issue, and Charles would help me solve it, giving me the tools and confidence to approach it in a caring but effective way. This day, exhausted by the emotional events at work, I needed Charles's advice, coaching, and probing questions to help me see the answers I desperately needed. Instead, I got a blank face looking back at me.

Charles and I often had our best conversations on our walks through the neighborhood or eating out at our favorite spots.

In the 1980s, Charles would help me solve the various problems I faced while in my first management job. With a small staff of three, you might think I'd have found it easy, but I still came up with a variety of predicaments for him to help me solve: One staff member wasn't as motivated as I would have liked. Then a personal drama developed between two other staff members, which negatively affected their working relationship. Another employee came to work over a half hour late—multiple times. Charles taught me skills to better protect my staff's self-esteem while addressing the improvements needed in their performance.

I was a go-getter and believed in the adage "It's better to ask for forgiveness than permission." I would then need Charles to coach me on smoothing some of the feathers I'd occasionally ruffle when upper management wasn't quite ready for some of my innovative ideas.

In the early 1990s, he helped me set the stage for a smooth transition when I began my term as the national president for my professional association. "The past board meetings have been contentious," I said to Charles. "People keep staking their ground. Many aren't listening to others. How do I create a different environment?" He suggested, "Why don't you hand out the buttons you've seen me wear—'None of us is as smart as all of us'—at your first board meeting. That should set the right tone. Then ask the board members what they'd like to get out of the board meetings. From there, you can set up a new process for how the meetings will be run, which will encourage listening and foster better communication."

Our relationship had been built on learning from each other—we always shared problems and discussed issues. He communicated tremendous wisdom and caring, especially regarding relationships. We didn't just skim the surface; we dove deep. That was what originally drew me to Charles and kept me intensely in love with him—the depth of our conversations coupled with deep respect.

So when this latest crisis with my staff took place, it suddenly hit me: My mentor was gone. I'd lost Charles. I felt empty and alone. At that moment, I began to grieve as if Charles had already died.

With this dreadful realization, I decided that I needed to read a book on grief to help me through. I borrowed a few books from the hospice social worker. Most tended to be about the intense struggle of losing a loved one. But I didn't want to wallow in grief; I wanted to read something that would give me courage. I wanted confidence that I could make it through this black hole.

I found the most help and support from a book my mother had given me earlier in Charles's disease. *Getting to the Other Side of Grief: Overcoming the Loss of a Spouse* gave me hope and comfort

with its positive viewpoint. "You will get to the other side," authors
Susan Zonnebelt-Smeenge and Robert De Vries wrote encouragingly.
The book helped me pinpoint what I missed about Charles. The
authors' probing questions helped me explore my feelings about this
awful loss:

- What did I value most about our relationship?
- What special memories do I have of my spouse?
- What will I take with me as a part of my spouse and our
  relationship to cherish?

I took a few nights to ponder my answer for each question. All of
my answers revolved around Charles's mentoring and support of me
as a person and of my efforts. The answers I found helped me hold
on to what I valued from our relationship. And defining what I'd lost
helped me to grieve.

Caregiving Affirmation:
It's perfectly normal to grieve even before your loved one dies.

PREPARING FOR THE INEVITABLE

I couldn't tell how long Charles would live, but his death started
to feel imminent. It was early 1999, and Charles appeared to be fading rapidly. His diminishing speech, his yelling, and his discomfort
seemed to be clues.

I felt that I needed to make preparations for his death, so I enlisted the help of my sister Carolyn on one of her visits. We contacted a
local funeral home to make arrangements for cremation. I met personally with the director and provided the information he needed. I
even took the time then to provide the content for Charles's obituary. I didn't want to feel pressured to do that in what I thought
would be his very hectic last days. For the obituary, I gave the director the names of three agencies for memorial gifts—the Employee
Ownership Foundation, the Society for PSP, and Wayside Hospice. I
also provided the director with the first part of Charles's mission
statement that he recited to himself every day. I told him that I
would pay whatever was needed to have the newspapers include it. I
wanted people to know the man Charles was.

Carolyn did research and found a person who could perform an autopsy on Charles's brain, and she documented the details of what we would need to do immediately upon his death to prepare for the autopsy. And she also worked with the Harvard Brain Tissue Resource Center (http://www.brainbank.mclean.org/) at McLean Hospital (http://www.mclean.harvard.edu/) in Belmont, Massachusetts, to understand the procedures for donating the autopsied brain for research.

Charles and I never talked about donating his brain. When he could still communicate, I had been afraid that he would interpret my bringing up the topic as meaning that I was eager for him to die so that I could move on with my life. But by the time the conversation became a necessity, he couldn't talk or communicate his wishes. I was convinced that I wanted science to have his brain, and I think he would have agreed. His type of disease is quite rare, so the research that could be done regarding the changes in his brain cells could possibly help others—another way for him to leave a legacy.

I took the time to also make a list of the people to be notified when he died. After checking off the family members and friends to include from our small address book, I typed up the names to have the list ready on its own sheet of paper. That would allow me to pass the unpleasant task of making the calls to another family member willing to help—and to make sure that no one was forgotten.

Hospice also provided me with information, and my mom passed along a checklist from her church of tasks that would need to be done.

From all of the tips that I gathered and prepared, I made a master to-do list. That's how I function day to day—I can't live without my to-do list. And I suspected that I might not be thinking clearly when Charles was dying, so I wanted to do as much of the preparation in advance as possible. This list would ensure that things wouldn't be forgotten.

First I organized the tasks to be done immediately after Charles's death, and worked with hospice to determine who would be responsible for each item. This included names and phone numbers, and was in chronological order:

- Call Brain Tissue Resource Center when death is imminent
- Call hospice to pronounce death
- Call funeral home to pick up body
- Call Carmen to do autopsy
- Get Dr. Ravin to complete death certificate
- Call church to set up date and time for memorial service
- Call list of friends and family to be notified

I did all of that sad organizing without emotion. Somehow I could separate the feelings of losing Charles from the task of preparing to lose him. I never let myself stop to think about what all of this really meant—that Charles was going to die soon. I'd gotten through a distasteful task in my exercise physiology lab in graduate school in the same way. We had to learn to draw blood from someone's arm. I had been ridiculously afraid of needles all of my life to that point. I didn't know how I was going to perform the skill well enough to pass the practicum. On my first practice try, I decided not to think about what I was doing—sticking a needle into someone's arm. Instead, I focused just on the steps to be taken and managed to get through without any emotion interfering.

Now was also the time, I thought, to make sure that people had a chance to see Charles to say good-bye. I encouraged his brothers to visit, and each one did. Many of my family members made it a point to travel to visit him. And we enjoyed seeing out-of-town friends, such as Kathryn from the study group in Charles's executive MBA program.

By June of that year, while Charles's mother was already in a nursing home for late stages of Alzheimer's Disease, his dad was dying of colorectal cancer. Ken, Charles's youngest brother, worked with the nursing home to obtain the medications, catheter, and other equipment that they would need to travel by airplane from Arkansas to Boston. David, the other brother, flew in from Florida. We all spent a weekend together, with my mom also visiting. At the end of the weekend, his eyes and his face ashen, Charles's dad spent time alone at Charles's bedside, saying his final good-bye. His dad died only three weeks after that trip.

During that visit with Charles's family, I finally executed a health care proxy. In Massachusetts, this form, like a living will, allowed

Charles to designate who would speak for him in a medical emergency. I had had the ominous blank document in my possession for quite some time. I hadn't been comfortable bringing it up with Charles—because of the same concerns I'd had about discussing the donation of his brain.

But with both brothers around, I got validation that this was the right thing to do, and they witnessed my signature. I even signed a health care proxy for myself, so that as we described this process to Charles, I would feel better that he wouldn't misinterpret my intentions. I learned one lesson: It would have been so much easier for us to have both filled out a health care proxy or living will many years earlier when we were both healthy. The importance of this was recently witnessed in the Terri Schiavo case.

I had made all the mundane preparations for his death and felt comfortable that the important people in his life had said their good-byes. There was only the uncertainty of how much time Charles had left.

Caregiving Affirmation:
Ease your burden by planning ahead for your loved one's death.

MOVE ON OR HANG ON?

I remember clearly the dilemma that hit me in October, when I was meeting with Kathleen, my new hospice social worker.

On one hand, I was beginning to feel like I wanted to move on with my life. For over four years, I'd been Charles's caretaker. I had started to feel that my life was on hold. Charles had lost all ability to communicate. He couldn't participate in life except by listening. We were no longer building our relationship together but were just waiting for it to wind down.

While I felt satisfaction in caring for Charles and making the best of his remaining time, it didn't seem like there was much to give him now. He was just existing—and it felt as if I was doing the same. And I was exhausted. Managing the responsibilities of the caregiving as well as working full-time had finally worn me out.

On the other hand, I still wanted to hang on to Charles. I didn't want to lose him from my life. For me to be able to move on, he would have to be gone—forever. I didn't really want that. Or did I? Was I ready for Charles to die? And it scared me to think about what life would be like without him. Was I ready to face that?

Of course, I couldn't do anything to make the situation progress any faster than it was. But I had no more physical or emotional energy for hanging on. I was mentally preparing for the next stage in my life as a result of the fatigue of working through the current stage.

Kathleen assured me that this conflict was normal.

But I couldn't move on just yet, because a new opportunity to promote Charles's book, *Paradoxes of Leadership*, was starting to emerge. Ever since the book was published, I had felt responsible for promoting it. With the help of his employee ownership friends, we had succeeded in popularizing it throughout the employee ownership community. Things had stalled as of late, so it was important to capitalize on this new chance.

Cal, Charles's friend from Web who accompanied us to Russia, had recently returned from his second trip to that country. He went with a Framingham contingent that had a sister city there. On the trip, Cal met Erica Mash, who wrote a weekly column for the local newspaper, the *MetroWest Daily News*. On returning, Cal suggested I talk to Erica about ways to solicit newspapers to write an article about Charles and his book.

Erica gave me the name of an editor at the *MetroWest Daily News*, and I promptly sent a letter requesting an interview for an article on Charles. To my surprise, the editor called and coordinated a time for the interview and to take pictures. I found out later that Erica had not yet had a chance to talk to the editor about Charles, so the interview request actually came on the merits of Charles's story.

The evening of the interview, Darry and I dressed Charles in his blue-and-white-striped golf shirt, my favorite. The photographer arrived and took pictures of the two of us, with Charles lying in his bed. The reporter came shortly after and interviewed me about Charles. He also talked to Darry.

The article, published on November 5, 1999, featured Charles on the front page of the paper's Life section. The headline read TRI-

UMPH OF THE SPIRIT, with our picture to the side. Bob Tremblay, the reporter, had captured the essence of Charles as well as of his book. He started the article, "To say the story of Charles R. Edmunson is inspiring is like calling Michelangelo's *Pietà* just a block of marble." The next paragraph set the stage:

> *In his book,* Paradoxes of Leadership, *Edmunson outlines his philosophy of life and work where empowerment and compassion are the cornerstones. A gifted speaker, skilled writer and successful executive who once ran nearly 2,000 days in a row as part of his routine, Edmunson now spends most of his time in a wheelchair unable to speak, write, read, walk and care for himself.*

The article described Charles's disease, his dedication to writing his book, and what life was like for him at the time of the interview. The article concluded:

> *What made Charles special as a leader, according to Janet, was that he practiced what he preached. "He cared about the people he worked with," she says. And it's now clear the feeling is being reciprocated. Unlike the book, there's nothing paradoxical about it.*

Getting this marvelous article in the local paper gave me confidence that Charles's legacy would be preserved—and ensuring that was becoming my passion.

Erica had also provided me with names of editors of the *Boston Globe's* West Weekly section. They, too, responded to my letter and published a touching article. The section front carried a large color picture of Charles and me. The photographer had taken the picture on an unusually warm late-November afternoon. We had rolled Charles in his wheelchair out onto the driveway, where autumn leaves graced the ground. I love the picture. It captures me gently caressing him while he, with his eyes closed, warms his face in the sun.

The story's headline honored Charles: EDMUNSON: 'A HEART WITH TWO LEGS.' Marty Carlock, the reporter, must have told the copy

editor who wrote it that Donnie Romine, president of Web
Industries, said that that was how another company officer described
Charles. And under the picture, there was a pull quote from June
Sekera, a close employee ownership friend of Charles's:

> *He is a Ghandi-esque person. He's a remarkable person who's
> had an enormous and always positive effect on everybody he's
> touched. The book is him.*

The rest of the article celebrated the contribution that Charles
and his book have made to the lives of others.

Both of these newspaper articles gave me confidence to press on.
I found out from the National Center for Employee Ownership, the
organization that published his book, that a Borders bookstore in
Framingham had ordered about fifteen copies. I assumed that it
occurred because of the local newspaper articles. I thought that it
might now be time to contact them to pursue a book signing with
Charles. I e-mailed Erica, with whom I was developing a friendship,
to see what she thought. To my surprise, she knew the woman who
coordinated all the events at Borders. Erica made an introductory
call, so that when I finally talked to the coordinator, she only asked
me, "When would you like to do it?"

Then I began to wonder: Was I taking on too much? I had been
living in a state of overwhelming exhaustion. Charles was nearly
bedridden. Was this worth the effort?

In addition, Charles's hospice nurse questioned whether this was
the right thing to do for Charles. Would this put him in an awkward
and embarrassing position? Was I being insensitive to his need for
dignity? Would he be a spectacle at the event? I respected her concern, but after some careful thought about these issues, I realized that
Charles's passion in life was to make a difference. This book signing
would provide a unique opportunity for him to continue to make
that difference. But because of the nurse's concerns, I tried to do
everything possible in the process to maintain his dignity.

Because Charles could no longer talk, I knew that I would have
to be the one to make the presentation. And I asked Loren, who

helped Charles write the book, to speak. We worked together to plan the outline for the presentation. Meanwhile, I searched Charles's old papers for one of his beautiful signatures. Charles, of course, couldn't sign books, so I went to an office supply store to get a stamp of his signature made. We would literally sign the books for him.

The book signing also gave me a chance to encourage Ken, Charles's younger brother, to come back up and visit. Ken had been the caregiver for their father and mother when both were sick; they had died within one week of each other in June of the previous year. After that, Ken would call us each week, but just couldn't work up the enthusiasm to visit us—it was just too painful for him to think of seeing Charles deteriorating. This event, though, provided the impetus for him to visit.

As the date for the book signing approached, I began to panic about whether Charles could physically handle the day. He had been getting quickly uncomfortable in his wheelchair. When that happened, he would let everyone know. And he had no control of his urinary tract or bowels. But I relaxed a bit when I realized that with lots of preparation, we would make it through. I developed contingency plans, including having Darry attend, along with the aide we had that day, just in case Charles didn't make it emotionally or physically. With their help, Ken would be able to take Charles home early if necessary.

On the day of the book signing, which was set for the early afternoon, Bobby was Charles's aide. He prepared Charles as usual for his daily activities—giving him a sponge bath, washing his hair in bed, and feeding him breakfast. I had all of our supplies packed and ready to go—tissues, moistened wipes, beanbag and other pillows, afghan, and extra Depends pads, as well as all of the book-signing materials, such as the signature stamp, printed sheet of Charles's paradoxes, extra copies of the book, camera, and my notes.

Figuring that we would have difficulty getting Charles into the car (he hadn't been in the car for about a year), I scheduled the RIDE (Massachusetts' transportation service for the handicapped; http://www.mbta.com/traveling_t/disability_theride.asp) to pick him up. That day, the RIDE came early and caught us off guard. We scrambled to finish getting Charles ready and in his wheelchair, and then loaded him into the van.

I had even visited Borders ahead of time to request a special sofa for Charles to sit on. There was one upstairs, but the book signing was going to be downstairs. My contact wasn't sure that the store could accommodate us. I was thrilled when we arrived on the day of the book signing to see that someone had placed a comfortable sofa in front, next to the lectern and facing the audience.

Most of the people present were Charles's or my friends and colleagues—people from Web Industries, the employee ownership community, the leadership program at Boston College, the company where I worked, as well as other dear friends. Nearly fifty people attended. Beginning the session, I spoke about Charles's work history at Web Industries, recounting how he'd started at the bottom as a packer, putting finished products into boxes for shipping. I described his rise to vice president of manufacturing and the lessons in leadership that he had learned along the way. I shared the expanded influence he had throughout New England, the nation, and even the world, spreading the word about the values of employee ownership and people-centered leadership.

Loren told the audience about how he had helped Charles with the process of writing his book. He also talked about some of what he called *Charles-isms*. His favorites were "No one sets out to be a jerk" and "We are emotional beings before we are rational beings." Then Loren and I read selections from our favorite chapters of the book, thanked people for coming, and stamped Charles's signature in their books.

Afterward, people talked about how touching it was to watch Charles—sitting in front on the comfy sofa with an afghan draped over his body—look intensely at Loren and me when we talked. I was quite moved watching Ken sit next to Charles and stroke him tenderly to keep him calm.

I realized after the book signing, though, that in the rush to get him ready for the event, I'd forgotten to give him his pills to help keep him calm and comfortable. Without the pills, our risk of a disaster erupting were multiplied. Knowing that, I felt even more fortunate that Charles made it peacefully through the event.

And I hoped that he understood what was going on in honor of him. Charles's powerful physical presence made this opportunity work and allowed us to fulfill the goal of preserving his legacy. Charles and I still had a mission to accomplish!

Caregiving Affirmation:
As long as your loved one hangs on,
look for reasons to hang on too.

TAKING CARE OF ME

As an extrovert, I needed regular contact with people, which was why continuing to work had been so important to me. But for the last year, I'd spent my weeknights with only Charles and the aide. Now, because I had enough help with Charles, I began to explore ways to be with friends and to better take care of my own needs.

SEEING FRIENDS

My longtime friend Jean made an effort to see me regularly. Once every couple of weeks, we met on a weeknight at a Framingham seafood restaurant to talk and have our shrimp, jasmine rice, and broccoli dinner. Jean understood my time constraints, so she made the forty-five-minute trip to my town instead of meeting me halfway as was our practice before Charles became ill. How long I had needed this kind of companionship! I unloaded about the latest issues with Charles, and work. Jean was a good listener and told animated stories that made me laugh. Occasionally we switched venues and met in West Newton to have a quick Italian meal—pasta with marinara sauce and vegetables—and see an independent film at the local theater there.

I made time for getting together periodically with Melanie, Arlene, and other friends, getting out one night a week. And I'm thankful for my old high school friend, Maureen, who called me just about every Sunday night and made me feel a part of life. I so needed that connection with my friends. And I discovered later that this reconnection ensured that my friends would know to be there when I really needed them during Charles's last days, and after he died.

GETTING EMOTIONAL AND PSYCHOLOGICAL SUPPORT

When I mentioned the yelling and other changes in Charles to the social worker that hospice had arranged for me to see, she recommended that I create a "love box."

"Put all of the letters you have saved from Charles and other memorabilia into it," she said. I didn't. But I did pull out and read the notes and letters that Charles had saved from when we first started dating. I began to remember anew his love, which he hadn't been able to verbalize to me for quite some time. Reading them now comforted me.

I also shared with the social worker my fear that I might be setting myself up for an emotional crash by having taken on such a heavy load myself. I thought that I might be deluding myself in thinking I was doing okay, and that maybe I would just lose it one day—as in post-traumatic stress syndrome. But she reaffirmed my coping skills, saying that she didn't think I would suddenly sink into the depths of depression. And, she said, "If you did, Janet, you would have friends and family that would recognize it and support you." This gave me confidence and reassured me that I truly was coping well, and would be able to make it through everything to come.

HAVING TIME FOR ERRANDS

In addition to the social worker, hospice provided extra aides to cover the weekends. That gave me time for whatever I wanted or needed to do for a few hours on a Saturday or Sunday. I no longer needed to scramble to get errands completed, and I'd have time to see a movie or enjoy a relaxing restaurant meal alone. I appreciated even the little things that hospice provided, such as the nurse's taking over the duty of filling Charles's pillbox each week. Before she did so, I had dreaded that task each time the last day's pills were emptied.

EXERCISING AGAIN

Over the previous couple of years, my exercise routine had suffered as I assisted Charles with his. We ran together, arm in arm, for as long as he could. But he went so slowly, I'm not sure how much exercise it actually provided me. Then we switched to walking together, until that became impossible to do. Now I could get back into my own independent exercise routine. But I felt guilty. Initially, I would head for the streets to jog while Charles was still in bed in the morning. I suspected that he was disappointed he couldn't go.

The actual jogging felt weird and frightening at first. My legs didn't feel like they would go. I didn't have complete control of them; they somehow felt detached from me. Terrified, I wondered if that was just what it felt like to be totally out of shape. Or was this something worse? Could I, too, be getting a neurological disease? Maybe multiple sclerosis or amyotrophic lateral sclerosis? But I just kept jogging to see if it would go away on its own. It took a year before I began to feel normal.

When I talked to Mickey, a friend of mine in medical school, he thought it might be psychomotor retardation, which is related to depression. It sounded reasonable to me because I did feel physically retarded when I was jogging. Wouldn't the fact that I had not been jogging for over a year and had been experiencing extreme fatigue and mental stress be a reasonable cause? However, when I talked later to Charles's neurologist after he died, she wondered if it could have potentially been something more serious and requested I see her if it happened again. But it never did.

As time went on, my sister Carolyn suggested that I not leave Charles alone while I was out on my jog, just in case something happened to him. And because I jogged early in the morning, before the aide arrived, I needed to come up with a new solution. I persuaded some of Charles's visiting male friends to lug the treadmill up from the basement and put it in our bedroom. I started using it every morning. While I would have preferred to run outside, I was thankful to Charles's ESOP friends for giving him the treadmill a few years earlier. Now it was finally being put to good use.

SETTING ASIDE TIME TO BE WITH MY LOVE

I started a Saturday-night ritual with just Charles and me. After the daytime aide left, I ordered a takeout tandoori chicken pizza on whole-wheat dough and rented a movie. After we finished eating the pizza, I'd bring out some double-fudge brownie low-fat frozen yogurt, and we'd share it right from the carton. Charles couldn't follow the movie and seemed disinterested in anything except the food. However, I looked forward to this weekly event.

HANDLING THE HOLIDAYS

For the upcoming Christmas holiday, Charles couldn't buy me gifts. He couldn't even ask about what I might want, so I started buying some clothes for myself from catalogs. When they arrived, I asked Mom, who was visiting, to wrap them for me. I was surprised that I had forgotten much of what I'd ordered when I opened them at Christmas.

Caregiving Affirmation:
Don't feel guilty taking some time for yourself;
you need it to stay healthy.

REFLECTIONS

Difficult experiences teach us precious lessons of wisdom. At this late point in dealing with Charles's disease, I had learned quite a few lessons:

Don't wait too long to get help. Trying to do it all seemed like the only way at first, but that eventually wore me down. I hadn't thought that Charles would accept help from home health aides—especially female ones. In retrospect, I found that once he had the help, he quickly got used to it, after a bit of complaining. I ended up missing out on needed help earlier in his disease.

Stress makes you stupid. I couldn't concentrate, couldn't find the right word I wanted, or I would just forget things. I understand that there is actually a physiological explanation for this phenomenon: Stress can impact our ability to think clearly. I was glad to realize that I wasn't really losing my mind.

Surround yourself with positive people and messages. I felt uplifted when I listened to the Norman Vincent Peale tape we had ordered for Charles through the National Library of Congress. I can't remember the names of the books on tape, but Peale's affirming theme of "You can if you think you can" gave me courage and assurance that my positive attitude was what would get me and Charles through. Two other quotes from Peale also encouraged me: "It's always too soon to quit" and "To every disadvantage there is an advantage." I wrote each of those down and kept the notes handy. They fit in well with a saying I had always tried to follow: "When life gives you lemons, make lemonade." With positive people and messages around me, I had the confidence to make it through this unimaginable life difficulty.

Strength comes in helping someone else. The more I committed myself to helping Charles fulfill his goals, the stronger I felt in my caregiving. I guess that was because I had become a partner with him in preserving his legacy, which provided meaning and purpose for this struggle.

It's difficult dealing with the very long good-bye that is part of a neurodegenerative disease. While I didn't hear her say this, I understand that Nancy Reagan used these words to describe living with Ronald Reagan's Alzheimer's disease. While I chose to be optimistic and tried to make the best out of our situation, I had nonetheless been losing my beloved Charles bit by bit. And that was still very difficult and painful.

Assisted suicide is probably not necessary. Earlier in Charles's disease, I had pondered whether assisted suicide might actually be a humane way for Charles to end his life, if living it was too difficult for him. If he was no longer contributing to life—and was just existing—why shouldn't we be allowed to do it? But I had learned that for Charles, even though he couldn't talk, he was still making an impact in others' lives. Even the hospice staff and volunteers, who had never heard him speak, commented on the powerful influence he quietly had on their lives. And because he didn't show that he was in too much pain, allowing nature to take its course seemed to be the right thing for us.

Be more upfront. I wish I could have dealt earlier with certain issues that arose with Charles, such as his driving, retirement, and getting a wheelchair. I felt that he needed to be emotionally ready to address some of these things. However, in some instances, I might have waited longer than I really should have. I found that I was able to get up the gumption to deal with potentially contentious issues only if I psyched myself up first. But even then, these issues took me out of my comfort zone. I watched for the appropriate opportunity and pounced on it when it came; in retrospect, I wish I could have been more proactive.

Life isn't fair. That was just the way it was. By accepting that life isn't fair, I was usually able to stay clear of the anger and frustration that can paralyze caregivers. My brother explained to me once that the Chinese symbol for crisis is danger plus opportunity. The danger just happened—Charles had a degenerative disease. Even though it was unfair, this tragic opportunity allowed me to live more deeply and passionately.

Caregiving Affirmation:
A positive attitude can help get you through the toughest times.

6

🌿

2000: Winding Down

FOCUSING ON PALLIATIVE CARE

During this stage of the caregiving, we focused on palliative care, hygiene, and avoiding pain, and not as much on keeping Charles entertained. This was a challenge because he couldn't communicate, but I am happy that we did the best we could.

Each morning, an aide drew warm water in the pink plastic pail. The aide then grabbed the bottle of Johnson's Baby Bath and a washcloth. It was time for Charles's bed bath. We had decided that it was no longer safe to shower him. A bed bath took about an hour, but the aide could safely and thoroughly wash him from head to feet. I found it interesting to see how the aide washed his hair while he was still in bed. The aide propped his shoulders and neck on a number of pillows, with his head extending beyond. With a pail of water under his head and some shampoo handy, the aide used the washcloth to work up the lather and then to rinse.

Once he was cleaned and dressed, the aide moved him into the wheelchair using the Hoyer lift. Dianne, the hospice nurse, declared that it wasn't safe anymore to lift Charles for the transfer like we used to do. His body was too limp, forcing us to lift completely dead weight.

A number of months earlier, Deedee had often asked me if we could get a Hoyer lift. Even though I had heard about the ease of using this lift at an earlier PSP support group meeting, for some reason I resisted. I don't know if I just didn't think it would be helpful, or if I didn't want another piece of handicapped equipment to crowd the house. We already had a wheelchair, recliner, and hospital bed with side table. One more piece of equipment just seemed like too much. But eventually I started to struggle to transfer Charles from his bed to his wheelchair by myself. That meant that when I was alone with Charles every Saturday and Sunday after 4:00 PM, he was stuck in his bed.

Now the Hoyer lift allowed me to move him again without too much difficulty and made life more comfortable for Charles by providing him with more options of places to sit or recline. To use the lift, I only needed to roll Charles from side to side, rather than lift him, to place the red canvas sling underneath him. Then after attaching the hooks at the end of cables to each corner of the sling, I would turn the crank, and the hydraulic system easily lifted Charles off the bed. He'd float in the air as I wheeled the lift in front of the wheelchair or recliner. I'm surprised he never yelled or seemed afraid to be hanging there in limbo. Once he was safely in place, I would simply turn the crank to lower him onto his next resting place. What an amazing device.

For the times when Charles was in the wheelchair, we had a system for keeping him from toppling over: We padded him with pillows on his right and left sides and buckled him in with a sort of seat belt.

His fingers continued to be clenched and stiff—looking deformed like those of my grandfather, who had had Parkinson's disease. We had to place a dry washcloth on his palms to keep his fingernails from cutting into his hands. However, we couldn't open his fists with brute force, because it would cause him excruciating pain. Instead, a hospice nurse taught us to hold his thumb with one hand and his fingers with another and gently pry the fist open. It worked every time.

Also, his arms bent rigidly at the elbow. Sores had begun to develop in the crease because no air hit that area. To clear them up and prevent them from coming back, we cleaned and dried them during his sponge bath and rubbed them with Gold Bond powder. Then as he sat in the wheelchair, we'd gently unflex his elbows and stuff pillows there to keep his arms straighter and drier.

Charles no longer looked like he used to. Not only did his arms and hands look deformed, but now his head tilted backward most of the time. The sides of his mouth puckered in. And his eyes looked out longingly like those of a baby waiting for his mother's care. The memory of this image hit me powerfully just after Charles died. When I looked into the eyes of a friend's baby, I choked back tears, as they reminded me so much of looking into Charles's eyes.

Feeding Charles had become trickier, too. We needed to stick mostly to soft foods, such as Jell-O and pudding. Then something very scary started to happen. Sometimes when we fed him, he seemed to fall asleep with his eyes open, and food that wasn't fully chewed or swallowed got stuck in his mouth. He just zoned out. We couldn't arouse him even when we'd shake him. Dianne suspected that the culprit was a seizure of some kind. He'd eventually "wake up" and miraculously begin chewing again. Unfortunately, these episodes became more and more frequent.

It also seemed as if he might have forgotten how to drink using a straw. He just wasn't sucking in the liquids. We tried using a toddler's sippy cup, holding it up to his lips and letting gravity drip the liquid into his mouth. This worked some of the time, but seemed to cause more coughing than the straw had.

Charles slept most of the time, listening off and on to the TV or music. We'd rotate him throughout the day between the recliner, bed, and wheelchair to give him variety and to protect him from bedsores.

But even at that, we couldn't prevent a mild sore that developed over his tailbone. We worked hard, coached by Dianne, to clear it up using a special cream and dressing. Because he'd lost so much weight and was now quite bony, other areas of his body began to look vulnerable to sores, so Dianne ordered him a unique air mattress. Its pump pushed air into some of the two-inch pockets on the surface of the mattress for about thirty seconds, then deflated those and filled others. By deflating and inflating different parts of the mattress, it rotated the pressure points for Charles, without our having to move him. All of the red spots vanished with this remarkable mattress.

At that point, our weekend aides from the agency were immigrants from Uganda. As we took Charles for a walk down the street in his wheelchair and talked, I learned a lot about this African country and its brutal past. Happily, I found these aides to be caring and conscientious—and great companions for both Charles and me. As we walked the streets of our neighborhood, I also enjoyed seeing some of my neighbors who would step out to say hello.

Charles's bowel movements still caused him problems. A couple of times, a movement caught an aide off guard and seeped through the Depends pad and leaked onto the carpet from his wheelchair. To clean up, we had to use a wet towel, Resolve carpet cleaner, and then a spray made to remove dog odors. His bowel movements were infrequent and sporadic, which made him frequently uncomfortable. And when they came, he cringed in pain—I believe because of an annoying hemorrhoid. I would be delighted when a bowel movement finally occurred. My mom found it amusing when she heard me cheer for joy, then saw me glove up for the cleanup. I was happy at his relief.

Unfortunately, other bothersome problems developed. His mouth and eyes became quite dry. We started a regular regimen of dropping artificial tears into his eyes and spraying artificial saliva into his mouth.

Then there were the scary episodes of shortness of breath that sometimes lasted as long as thirty minutes. One of the on-call hospice nurses thought it might be a vagal stimulation response, which is the result of something pressing on the vein that brings blood back to the heart from the body. She said that this could happen if Charles pushed too hard to have a bowel movement, which often explained the situation. Charles usually calmed down as soon as I started to talk to a hospice nurse on the phone or when I gave him some liquid morphine, as the nurses instructed me to do.

Brushing Charles's teeth became nearly impossible. At first he started biting down on the toothbrush, making it difficult to dislodge. We'd have to wait until he finally loosened his jaw and let it go. After I talked to my dentist, I ordered a child-size bite block for Charles. It was a piece of black rubber about an inch square. We tied a string around it so we would always be able to pull it out. Charles bit down reflexively on it—hard. But the small opening it created allowed a brief opportunity to get a toothbrush inside his mouth.

On Saturdays, Stacey arrived at 10:00 AM to give Charles a massage. If she was lucky, he would lie comfortably and not squirm. With peaceful music playing, Stacey soothingly worked his weakened muscles, mostly to pamper and relax him. Then, with his hour-long massage complete, the aide kept watch over him while Stacey and I went upstairs to one of our guest bedrooms. As I lay on my stomach with my head at the end of the bed, Stacey kneeled on the floor and for thirty minutes gently massaged the tight muscles in my upper back and neck, something my body truly needed but that I hadn't had time on my own to get. Although the massages were originally intended for Charles's relief, they calmed me even more than they did him.

Caregiving Affirmation:
Being able to provide only palliative care and not curative care
can feel scary, but know that you are doing the best
you possibly can for your loved one.

So Much Promise . . .

After Charles's mother and father died in June 1999, his brother Ken had located a stash of memorabilia in the musty den of his parents' run-down house. On Ken's last visit, he brought the box of items that his mother had collected throughout Charles's childhood, adolescence, and university years. Ken and I looked through the box together on his visit that fall. Charles couldn't talk at the time, and I'm not really sure how much he could understand. But in his presence, Ken and I delighted in reading the old report cards, science project awards, and yellowed newspaper articles on his academic and sports achievements.

I had always known that Charles was smart; he had told me he was valedictorian of his high school class in Arkansas. But it wasn't until Ken and I read through the items in this box that I realized just how intelligent he was.

We found the results of the standardized Iowa Test of Basic Skills that Charles took in the fourth grade. His total score of 98 meant that he did better than 98 percent of all fourth graders in America on all of the skills—vocabulary, reading, language, work-study, and arithmetic. Ninety-eight percent! That meant that he had not only excelled academically in a small high school in Arkansas, but also must have been one of the smartest kids in the entire country.

Charles's baby book, also in this box, showed some interesting firsts—waving good-bye at 7 months, saying his first words—*da-da-da* and *'bye*—at 7 3/4 months, and standing and walking at 9 1/4 months. I especially loved the picture of Charles at 10 1/2 months, with his chubby little body sitting on a shag rug, his nose scrunched up and his tongue sticking out between his four baby teeth. And the original birth certificate had his teeny footprints on the back, showing early evidence of the extremely wide forefoot he had as an adult.

After Charles left home, his mother saved a number of his letters. They chronicled his time at college in Tampa, Florida, and then the next few years when Charles, married to his first wife, went to Jackson, Mississippi, to preach, then returned to Tampa, and finally moved to Boston for graduate school.

From the college letters, a number of themes emerged. One was his concern about bothering his parents for money. I chuckled out loud when he wrote, "I have eighteen cents left out of that twenty dollars. Maybe it will last me the rest of the month." Other themes he consistently wrote about included his intense debate club activities, the racial prejudice he was surprised to witness among the religion school's professors and students, and always questions about how his brother David was doing with senior math and how Ken was doing with football.

The most poignant letter Charles wrote came during graduate school in Boston, apparently after he told his parents about his upcoming separation from his wife. He wrote, "I hope you're not upset at my not telling you sooner—it's *hard*. I love you—and I need you. But please don't *worry* about me. I'm going to be all right—eventually."

Lying in his bed, Charles didn't fidget as we rummaged through his past. From his lack of facial expression, we couldn't tell whether he understood what we were looking at or our excitement at learning so many wonderful and painful things about his past. I hoped he was proud that I was seeing some of his boyhood and young adult accomplishments. It pleased me to be examining these things with him looking on, instead of discovering them after he had died.

Ken and I read meticulously through that box—he remembering the past with Charles, me getting to know Charles better. It was bittersweet, seeing the hope of the past and then looking over at Charles in the present, devastated by this terrible disease. All of the items in the box showed so much promise for Charles in the future. Because of his disease, though, it would never be fully realized. But what a special privilege for me to be able to peer into Charles's life history and appreciate even more profoundly the person he was.

Caregiving Affirmation:
It's okay to mourn what might have been.

THE END IS COMING

"Janet, I'm so sorry to tell you this," Deedee said, "but I'm going to take a new job as a day-care teacher. I'll be starting in two weeks." Off and on over the last year or so, Deedee had mentioned that she was looking for a change. For a while, she thought about going back to school for a degree in psychology, but she'd finally settled on making a career change to teach preschoolers. Though this devastated me and, I suspected, Charles, I certainly understood. Deedee had cared for Charles for three years now. We all knew he was close to the end of his life. Deedee needed to move on. I'm certain that Charles would have supported her in this move and the opportunity for growth that it afforded her, had he been able to talk and comprehend the situation.

Hospice now took on the difficult task of looking for a new aide to cover the four weekdays that Deedee worked. "Janet, I'm still looking," Dorothy at hospice would say in her Irish accent. "I've got calls into three agencies. I'll let you know something when they call me back. It's not looking good yet, but something will work out." But even Dorothy's optimistic outlook and hard work couldn't solve this one. What had been a growing crisis in our area—a shortage of home health aides—had now become our problem. Dorothy couldn't find one person to cover all of Deedee's days, so we started to have a variety of new aides in and out of our home. Charles had unique issues that the aides would need to address, so I typed up instructions and prepared as much as I could in advance, readying clothes and meals for the day.

Then shortly after Deedee's announcement, Carlos, our early morning aide for the past two years, said one morning in his Brazilian accent, "Janet, I'm so sorry to tell you that I will be leaving you soon. I am going to work with my friend in his new carpet business." He explained that this opportunity promised to pay much more than working as an aide.

How would I cope with both Deedee and Carlos leaving at the same time? And Charles seemed to be slipping quickly into a deeper decline. I felt vulnerable facing the stormy waters ahead.

Caregiving Affirmation:
Expect the unexpected.

Then Mom arrived. Because of her church orchestra schedule, she came up a week before the date she'd originally planned. Her timing proved perfect. I'd never needed her more. With her helping out, I wouldn't have to leave Charles alone with new aides each day. Her presence allowed me to continue to work and gave me tremendous peace.

Mom and each new day's aide would be a good balance. Mom made sure the aide kept to Charles's special routine. She could also prepare the soft meals and thickened drinks Charles needed. But because Mom weighed only one hundred five pounds, the aide had to provide the muscle to keep Charles comfortable. Mom and I decided not to replace Carlos, but to instead have the day aides bathe Charles when they arrived. With Mom in the house, I didn't need to wait for the aides' arrival and could continue to go in to work at my usual time.

One day, hospice couldn't find an aide—the very day I *had* a pilot program at work starting with some area physician offices. I had to be there for this first day of the project, and it had been so complicated getting all the physician office visits scheduled for the project that I hated to postpone them. After that day, I could stay at home if it was absolutely necessary, but I was so grateful when Mom graciously agreed to care for Charles alone that day.

We worked on how she would use the Hoyer lift to move him into the recliner. And we practiced using the draw sheet underneath him to help her turn him over in bed. If using the Hoyer lift became too complicated, she could just leave him in bed for the day. However, she would need to clean him up if he urinated or had a bowel movement—no way to get around that messy and embarrassing task. But as unpleasant as that might be, she cheerfully convinced me that she was willing to do it—and in fact, she did.

I don't know if it was Deedee's leaving, the disruption of the strange new aides, or just the final weakening of his body, but it seemed that Charles had made the decision that it was time to go. I don't know if he made it consciously or unconsciously, but none of us questioned his intent. He just stopped eating. He clamped his mouth shut, and wouldn't take in any food.

"Not eating is natural," Dianne, our hospice nurse, assured us. "It will allow his body to quietly shut down."

That was what I wanted to hear. All throughout this disease I had had horrible fears about how Charles might die. People with PSP often aspirate (inhale into their lungs) their food or saliva and then get pneumonia and die. And my fears increased when Charles's dad, in the late stage of colon cancer, died of pneumonia. Ken, who cared for their dad through the entire ordeal, told me about the terror in his dad's eyes as he painfully suffocated with the pneumonia. Ken couldn't get the staff at the nursing home to increase the morphine enough to eliminate his dad's trauma.

"How long will it take for Charles to die?" I asked Dianne. "A few days to a week," she said. "We'll start giving him morphine whenever it looks like he needs it." I now had confidence that with hospice, I could handle the part of this disease that I had dreaded most—Charles's actual death.

SAYING GOOD-BYE

"Starting last Tuesday, May 2, Charles stopped eating and drink-

ing," I wrote as an attachment to the "thought for the week" e-mail I
sent. "We have been able, most of the time, to at least get his pills in
with some Jell-O. He is, however, very comfortable and peaceful. His
brother David has been visiting this weekend, and my mom is here
for a few weeks. We have been reading to Charles a lot of the letters
and tributes that many of you have given or sent to him in the past.
We continue to be struck by how much Charles seems to have
touched so many people's lives. This gives us great peace and comfort
and allows us to let him go."

This announcement, and calls I made to his close friends and
coworkers, served to alert people that it was time to say good-bye.
Over the next week, many visited—some alone, others in pairs—all
of them experiencing a sense of deep loss. I left them alone with
Charles. But when I saw the tears in their eyes as they left, I grieved
with them, in addition to grieving for my own loss. "It's like a
wake," my friend Melanie observed one day.

David, a deeply spiritual man, took the opportunity to say his
farewells and to pray with his brother.

Meanwhile, my mother and girlfriends provided me with needed
support and diversions. It was too difficult to focus only on all the
good-byes and Charles's impending death. Mom and I enjoyed the
almond-crusted goat-cheese salad one day for lunch at a restaurant
down the street. Melanie played Scrabble with Mom and me, and
Jean and Arlene visited.

E-mails for Charles came in as well. People from around the country shared their thoughts with Charles. I bawled with each one I
read, then wept again when I read them out loud to Charles.

- From Rob, a Web employee whom Charles had mentored: "I
  always believed that the highest amount of respect and love I can
  show Charles comes from going out into the world and truly living out the values and beliefs he helped me discover."

- From Bob, one of the general managers at Web, "I know that
  your life has touched hundreds and now through us will touch
  thousands more."

- From Bev, a woman who started at Web in Indianapolis as an
  administrative assistant: "Charles has had an enormous effect on

my life. He supported my desire to further my education and constantly told me, 'You are a learner, Bev.' I would like to tell
Charles that so far I have 103 college credits."

* From Michael, the new manager at one of Web's subsidiaries
and a friend of Charles's from the employee ownership community: "Please let Charles know that we continue to make progress at
FilmX on building the kind of company he would be proud of."

* From Ginny, a close employee ownership colleague: "I do
think of Charles often and he always serves as a quiet but persistent role model in my mind when I am wondering how to
approach something or someone or when I am feeling 'lost' in a
problem with someone. He gives me comfort and regularly
reminds me of the importance of 'grace.' "

Caregiving Affirmation:
You'll do friends and family members a kindness
if you invite them to say their good-byes—
but be prepared to mourn with them.

One morning, Charles started groaning. He kept letting out a
throaty "Mmmm," one right after another. This wasn't like any
noise in the past, so I called Dianne and asked what it could mean.
After she quizzed me regarding any signs of physical distress, which
I didn't see, she gave a potential explanation. "We sometimes notice
this in Alzheimer's patients. The thought is that they are dealing
with some unresolved emotional or spiritual stress," she said. After
I hung up the phone, I began to think about what issue might be
troubling Charles.

Kneeling down beside him and stroking his hair, I began to talk to
him. "Charles, you've made a tremendous difference in so many people's lives. We won't forget you. Your life has made an impact. I love
you, and I will always love you. I will also do everything possible to
keep you comfortable throughout this process. I'm not the best person to say this, as I don't think I believe in God. But if there is a
God, He will understand your searching and welcome you with open
arms. You can be at peace with this."

Almost immediately he stopped the groans and went calmly
to sleep.

HIS FINAL DAY

May 11. As soon as I woke up, I knew something was different.

Charles's breathing was heavy and labored. When I tried to roll
him over to the other side, to see if that would help, his whole body
went limp—like a sack of bones. He reminded me of the Holocaust
victims I had seen in pictures. I quickly laid him back into his earlier
position. His feet, lower legs, and fingertips felt cold to my touch.

I called Dianne, his hospice nurse, and she promised to come
right away. "Should I start to give the morphine now? Or wait until
you get here?" I asked.

"Start it now," she replied.

When she arrived at about 9:30 AM, she confirmed that she didn't
expect Charles to last the day. She needed to see other patients and
so wouldn't be able to stay, but she said to call hospice as soon as he
died, and she would come back. She said that meanwhile, I was to
give Charles the morphine every two hours.

Charles's original health aide, Gerard, on one of his frequent visits
to just see Charles, had begged me to make sure to call him if we
suspected his impending death. When I called that morning, though,
he wasn't home, so I gave the message to his wife.

My sister Sue fortuitously arrived from West Virginia early that
morning. She had planned to arrive later in the day but then decided
to drive the entire night. Once she saw Charles's deteriorating condition, she started calling family members and holding the phone to
his ear to allow them to speak to Charles. She hoped that that would
strengthen the connection between Charles and his family.

Stacey, his massage therapist, came as well. Bravely, she gave him a
full hour of healing touch and gentle massage of the head and feet,
her comforting music playing in the background.

My entire team from work visited late that morning. They came
to encourage me and to see Charles. My relationship with them goes
beyond just work; they're like family, and I felt thankful for their

presence. They had just the right words to say. Even after my warning that he was dying, courageously each one wanted to also see Charles and share their love.

For the entire day, we mostly kept Charles on his left side, as he seemed in less distress that way. When I had time alone with him, I read aloud the chapter on death from *The Prophet*, as well as some sections from *Luminata*, which Gigi, one of my staff members, had loaned to me.

The coldness that started in his feet and hands now moved up to cover his legs and arms, with his hands turning blue. Throughout the day, he breathed shallowly and rapidly. As the day progressed, he got into a pattern of fast breaths that then slowed, until he held his breath for a period, which I timed at about seven seconds. When he started to breathe again, his breaths began slow, then got fast, until the entire sequence repeated itself over and over again.

Gerard drove up at about 5:30 PM, which happened to be about ten minutes before Charles died. Darry had arrived for the evening shift, and Charles's friend Cal also had come by. Soon after Gerard entered the bedroom, Charles's breaths remained fast and became more labored. Gerard, a former nurse, announced, "This is it." I yelled for Sue and Mom, and we all gathered around Charles's bed, each touching him softly as Gerard coached us regarding what to expect next.

Charles stopped breathing for what seemed to be an eternity. Then he took one deep breath, then stopped again. Another deep breath. Then he stopped again before taking his final deep breath.

Charles died at 5:45 PM.

The end had a strange way of hitting each of us. I immediately sobbed. Once I recovered, Cal broke down, then later Darry. This allowed us all to comfort the one in pain.

With shaky hands, I dialed the number for hospice and told them of Charles's death. They immediately contacted Dianne, who was forty-five minutes away but would come as quickly as she could. Once Dianne arrived, she called the funeral home. Dianne completed the paperwork, and then the funeral home director took Charles away just after my giving him one last kiss and saying, "I love you."

At about 7:00 PM, I panicked when I remembered that the ESOP Association was holding its awards dinner in Washington, D.C. that night. I needed to contact someone there right away. Charles's close employee ownership friends would be getting together. And during the awards ceremony, the director would be giving out the Charles R. Edmunson Scholarships to the winners. These scholarships reflected the values that Charles brought to the organization—of honoring, rewarding, and recognizing others. I called the hotel frantically to locate the association president, Michael, before the program started. "You have to find him—my husband just died," I said in a quivering voice to the hotel recep-tionist. That wasn't exactly what I'd meant to say, but it got her attention, and she quickly found him.

Charles's ESOP friends related to me later that Michael waited until just after the awards ceremony to announce, "I'm sad to inform you that at 5:45 tonight, Charles Edmunson passed away." They said that many in the room sighed audibly in grief and then sat stunned at the timing of his death—with so many people who loved him gathered together. In Charles's honor, many of his closest friends hiked to the Thomas Jefferson Memorial that night and read the ESOP Association vision statement to Tom (Thomas Jefferson)—a tradition Charles started many years ago.

Just as Thomas Jefferson contributed many hours and his writing talent to craft the U.S. Constitution, Charles had worked all night a number of years ago to draft the vision statement for the association, a document that set a new course for the organization, as the Constitution did for America.

I was awed when I realized that Charles had died nearly five years to the day after he'd noticed the very first symptom of his disease—stumbling up and down the stairs of the Capitol building in Washington at the ESOP conference.

Caregiving Affirmation:
Don't hide from your loved one's death.
Open your heart to it, so that your loved one can let go
more easily and so that you can begin to grieve in earnest.

7

2000–2001: Grieving Made Easier by Promoting His Legacy

MISSION ACCOMPLISHED

I received tremendous support after Charles died. Family members flew in to Boston to help with all of the memorial arrangements—and most importantly, to be together to honor Charles.

I think Charles would have been pleased with the church in which we held the memorial service. He loved old buildings and would have appreciated the old church with its cozy feel and curved pews. We were not required to have a minister, so I planned a program to have speakers from all his major walks of life—his family, my family, and people from Web Industries, from Boston College's Leadership for Change program, and from the employee ownership community.

I served as host and coordinated the program, which was planned to include segments about Charles—his mentoring and touching people, leading by his paradoxes, spiritual searching, his humorous side, giving grace, and the impact of his love for me. Gigi, one of my staff members, sang the songs between the segments, including "Wind Beneath My Wings," "Because You Loved Me," and "Amazing Grace." The music powerfully stitched the program together. We finished the service with everyone reciting Charles's mission statement.

The service lasted two hours, with the speakers telling compelling and inspirational stories about Charles. It gave me peace to know that Charles had heard many of these accolades while he was still alive, and I relished having all those in attendance hear them. And many of the people commented to me on how the stories touched them. I created a newsletter to distribute during the service and to send to those who couldn't attend. It not only outlined the events of the service but also shared the story of Charles's life and displayed pictures of him and his endearing smile.

After the memorial in Boston, my mom and I flew to Arkansas to host a remembrance for Charles at his youngest brother's home in the town where Charles had attended high school. That allowed many members of Charles's extended family and old local friends to visit. We scattered some of his ashes at the graveyard where his mother and father were buried.

Later that spring, Boston College's Leadership for Change program invited me to share memories of Charles at the last event of the year, named after Charles, for its graduates. And since then, I've given my presentation about Charles at that final event every year. This provides me with yet another way to keep his legacy alive and to help Charles's life continue to affect others.

Caregiving Affirmation:
Soak up the precious tributes to your loved one,
who lives on through them.

THE WAVES—WHAT TOUCHES ME AND WHAT I AM LEARNING

All the experts say that grief comes in waves. They're right. And the size of the waves can be unpredictable. During the waves—triggered by a movie, song, book, letter, conversation, picture, or just a memory—the tears came. Sometimes just a single tear, other times sobs. But in the wave's wake, there was often comfort, learning, and encouragement. I began to welcome the waves and the release of emotion they brought.

MEMORIES AND PICTURES

I knew intellectually that Charles was dead, but it didn't feel real. I wrestled with the personal paradox that though I continued to feel Charles's very real presence, I missed him terribly. This was the source of most of my grief.

But grief flowed in from other sources, too. About two months after Charles's death, I suddenly experienced how Charles might have felt about being trapped in his body. I don't remember where I was when this wave hit. I hadn't had those types of thoughts before, being too wrapped up in my own experience of our plight. And I think I had engaged in wishful thinking, hoping that his dementia was strong enough to mask how ensnared he really was. But there it was. It flooded through my entire being. I felt as if I were on the inside of a nearly paralyzed body, looking out. I felt Charles's pain and despair at being locked in his body. With this stormy wave crashing on top of me, I was horrified.

For a few months after his death, I frequently relived his final day. I fixated on what I could have done differently and how he might have felt. Could I have comforted him more throughout the day? Had he been in pain? Had he needed more morphine? What was he thinking and going through? Was he afraid? What grief these painful thoughts brought me.

I did find more comfort than pain in looking at pictures of Charles, even photos taken once his disease became evident. I've displayed pictures of Charles and our friends and family everywhere, on my refrigerator, end tables, and bookshelves. I don't want to forget Charles or have his memory fade as time goes by. I read about a woman who decided to move out of her home almost immediately after her husband died because the house had too many memories of him. She felt she needed to move on. I suppose I'll get to where I'm ready to move on, but now, I feel comforted by these pictures of Charles. Over the next few years, these pictures comforted me. Now that I have remarried, I still have a special place in our home devoted to Charles, with pictures and memorabilia.

SONGS AND MOVIES

Tears released my pent-up grief like never before at the climactic ending of the suspense movie, *The Sixth Sense*. As we sat in the padded theater seats, my sister Barb just hugged me as my shoulders shook and I wept uncontrollably. The movie had been an illusion, with the main character believing he was alive, when he was really dead and living in the spiritual realm. I broke down at the very end when he finally recognized that he was dead. I then felt the terrific sorrow his wife had been expressing throughout the movie, grieving his death. Her pain was mine.

On another day, I was driving home alone from work when I heard Celine Dion's voice on the radio: "You are safe in my heart / and my heart will go on and on." The movie *Titanic* meant a lot to me when Charles and I saw it together midway through his disease. But the words of the movie's theme song hadn't caught my attention until that ride home—and I bawled the rest of the ride home. Hearing the song after Charles died put it all together for me. The main female character survived the sinking of the *Titanic*, and the man who caught her attention and helped her break free from the bonds of the English upper class drowned. She was able to start a new middle-class, yet meaningful, life in America. She recognized that her lover, although dead, was still an important part within her, and because of his brief but powerful influence on her life, she kept going. Even though the song continues to bring tears to my eyes, it reassures me that Charles's impact on my life allows me to go on, changed by his love and inspiration.

READING GRIEF BOOKS AND NEWSLETTERS

The waves of sorrow gently rolled over me when I read books on grief after Charles died. But that was their job, to help me process my grief and provide encouragement so that I could make it through. I reread some books that helped me earlier and picked up others that were new to me. Particularly supportive for me was a small paperback that a secretary from one of Charles's offices had sent with her sympathy card. *How to Survive the Loss of a Love,* by Bloomfield, Colgrove, and McWilliams, assured me that the pain

would heal. "You Will Survive," one page was titled. It then went on
to say:

> *You* will *get better.*
> *No doubt about it.*
> *The healing process has a beginning, a middle and an end.*
> *Keep in mind, at the beginning, that there is an end. It's not*
> *that far off. You* will *heal.*
> *Nature is on your side, and nature is a powerful ally.*
> *Tell yourself, often, "I am alive. I will survive."*
> *You are alive.*
> *You will survive.*

I waited until I had climbed into bed each night to read the sympathy cards I had received in the mail that day. This routine provided
a meaningful time for me to reflect on each card's message. And
though many brought me to tears as I pondered the loss of Charles,
they also encouraged me as I read how Charles had affected the card-
sender's life. Occasionally, though, a card would reflect on me and
how I'd supported Charles throughout his disease. Those were both
humbling and comforting. One card I read over and over came
from my sister Sue:

> *He'll always be remembered*
> *As a man, both strong and good,*
> *Who gave his best for others*
> *And who did the best he could.*
> *He'll always be remembered*
> *For all the joy he brought,*
> *As a man who made a difference*
> *And a man who meant a lot.*
>
> *Now as*
> *you remember*
> *the kind of caring ways*
> *Your loved one*

brought such happiness
into so many days . . .

May it bring
some consolation
to remember, too,
How many times
your loved one found
great happiness in you."

In addition to the messages of the cards themselves, the handwritten notes on the cards touched me in a personal way. The notes that meant the most to me mentioned Charles's gifts and presence, talked about the contributions I must have made to Charles and to us as a team, and acknowledged the special wisdom that life and death bring. But even cards without any personal notes meant a lot because I knew that people were thinking of me enough to take the effort to buy, address, and send a card. I've saved all of the cards, and I reread them occasionally. From my perspective, it's never too late to send a sympathy card. Even the ones that came a month or more after Charles's death encouraged me.

I took tremendous comfort from writing thank-you notes. I started a tradition by taking my note cards to Charles's favorite breakfast restaurant, Sunnyside Café, each weekend. I also wrote thank-you notes to people who supported me in special ways throughout his disease, spoke at his memorial service, or made charitable contributions in his name. Writing these notes allowed me time to remember what Charles (and I) meant to these people. After I'd finished all the thank-yous, I continued this tradition, breakfasting at the café and writing cards to friends and family to keep in touch.

The monthly bereavement guides from hospice also provided comfort. My favorite guide suggested writing down my thoughts, prompted by a list of issues to consider. I had already started writing this book, so I didn't write down my responses. Instead, I took one issue each night and thought about my response to that one issue.

This allowed me to remember Charles and talk to him, even though he was already gone.

The first prompt was "A special memory that I have about you . . ." That got me to remember the details of our tenth anniversary, when Charles shared the folder of notes from our first dates. The next prompt from the guide—"What I miss most about you . . ."—led me to remember the wonderful ways Charles had built me up and mentored me. "What I wish I had said or hadn't said . . ." hurt to think about. But my answer to it was that I wish I had said even more about how much Charles meant to me. The answer to "What I'd like to ask you . . ." came clearly to me. I asked Charles, "Did you feel supported by me through your death?" And my favorite issue to think about was "Ways in which you continue to live on in me . . ." *Lots*, I thought, and said, "Your influence on me as a leader and in caring for people. Also through the self-esteem that you helped me build and in who I am."

CONVERSATIONS

The psychiatrist with whom I'd worked on a postpartum depression project at work had not been aware, until after Charles died, that I was dealing with his illness. Seeing me shortly after my return to work, the psychiatrist asked, "Janet, do you have any regrets? Some people who work while caring for a dying family member have regrets." I immediately said, "No. I don't." And I honestly believed that. When I talked to the hospice social worker, Kathleen, about this, she said that I had actively cared for Charles even though I continued to go to work. "People who seem to have regrets are those who work more, travel more, and let other people deal with the caregiving."

But in reflecting about regrets now, I can think of a few. I wish I had called Charles every day from work and had the aide put the phone to his ear so that I could talk to him. I wish that after he could no longer talk, I had been more able in the evenings to carry on longer one-way conversations with him about what had happened that day at work. I wish I had stayed right by his side the entire day that he died. While I had a very special time with him that day, I started a lot of planning for the memorial service, instead of just sitting with him. But I knew that I needed to remember that such doubts plague most people dealing with the loss of a loved one. And when I process them now, I am sure that Charles always knew that I loved him, no matter what. That certainty helped an awful feeling of regret to subside.

Caregiving Affirmation:
Know that if you welcome the waves of grief
and the emotions that they evoke,
you are helping yourself to heal.

AUTOPSY REVEALS DIAGNOSIS

IT WASN'T PROGRESSIVE SUPRANUCLEAR PALSY

Seven months after Charles died, I finally received his brain autopsy report, which listed and documented two diagnoses: CBGD and mild to moderate cerebral arteriosclerosis.

Our primary neurologist, Dr. Paula Ravin, had suggested CBGD as a possible diagnosis early on. But after reviewing details of three years of Charles's symptoms and test results, the full neurological movement disorders team at a prestigious Boston hospital had declared that he had PSP. Charles's case clearly shows how difficult it is to get a diagnosis for these rare neurological conditions.

All along, though, I had feared that Charles might actually have CBGD. His symptoms fit the CBGD description quite well—and they were much worse and stranger than the PSP symptoms. And CBGD apparently progresses faster than PSP. As one article states, "The progression is relentless," which perfectly describes our experience. As I now reread the literature on CBGD, everything is so much clearer in hindsight.

Even though Charles had severe problems with his eye movements, his primary problem wasn't with looking down (called downward gaze), the symptom that is classic for PSP. His problems stemmed from an inability to move his eyes where he wanted to look, a lack of depth perception, a loss of peripheral vision, and choppy movement of his eyes in any direction.

Symptoms of CBGD usually start with marked rigidity on one side of the body. Charles's disease affected his right side first. The severity of the stiffness amazed even the doctors.

Apraxia also marks CBGD. Because of his apraxia, Charles's body would not respond to the movements he attempted, such as clapping his hands or touching a finger to his nose. He also described the weird sensation of his foot not feeling like a part of his body. Neurologists said that the sensation is alien limb phenomenon, another symptom more closely associated with CBGD.

In CBGD, speech is hesitant, movement is poor, and finding words is difficult—and Charles experienced all of these. Some articles we read reported depression and obsessive-compulsive symptoms, strongly apparent in Charles.

The autopsy finding of cerebral arteriosclerosis actually gave me some serenity because my reading led me to believe that cerebral arteriosclerosis can cause dementia. If this is indeed true, then I can take some comfort in the possibility that Charles wasn't completely cognizant during the extreme deterioration that ravaged his body and made him totally helpless at the end of his life. But paradoxically, I also hope he perceived the love and admiration we all felt for him, and that he was aware of our presence.

But perhaps the greatest comfort was in finally having the solution to the mystery that Charles and I had lived with for five years.

Caregiving Affirmation:
Consider an autopsy for your loved one to bring you peace of mind and the satisfaction of helping to further scientific knowledge.

NEW UNDERSTANDING OF CHARLES'S SYMPTOMS

I had a real hunger to better understand the brain autopsy report. I needed to comprehend the science behind it. Dr. Michael Gamache, a neuropsychologist, agreed to speak to me about Charles's report.

His insightful explanations helped me understand quite well how the disease process resulted in Charles's symptoms. He described how the higher part of the brain, through deterioration, became disconnected with the lower part of the brain. He explained that "the higher part, consisting partially of the frontal lobe of the brain, supplies the filter we use in controlling behavior. It is the executive part of the brain. It allows us to process the information we take in and determine what to do with it. It permits us to apply reason, weighing the pros and cons prior to making decisions and performing actions. The lower part of the brain provides us with sensory perception—such as feeling that something is hot or that a room is dark."

Dr. Gamache explained that in CBGD, the disconnect between the higher and lower parts of the brain clearly cause the symptoms of apraxia and alien limb phenomenon. Charles's brain knew what to do, but the connections from its higher part to its lower part had degenerated, which made it impossible for the signal to perform an action or perceive a feeling to get through.

"An emotional response of frustration and depression would be common for someone like Charles, who comprehended that he should be able to do something but then couldn't," Dr. Gamache said. That clearly described why Charles reacted to his unusual and disturbing symptoms with such frustration and sadness.

Dr. Gamache described that the autopsy report showed deterioration also of the actual neocortex, or higher part of the brain—not just of the connection between the higher and lower areas of the brain. Because the neocortex provides the filter and reasoning we use to control our behavior, we can lose inhibitions when it deteriorates.

To help me understand the functioning of the neocortex, Dr. Gamache described something that happened in 1848 to a railroad construction foreman, Phineas Gage. During construction of the railroad, Phineas hadn't cleared the area in time before some explosives went off. The explosion shot his tamping iron through the frontal lobe of his brain. He survived, but the accident caused a disconnect of the frontal lobe with the rest of the brain. Before the accident, he had been a calm, organized, and capable man. After the accident, he became disorganized and irritable and acted peculiar. The disconnect took away his self-restraint. (For more details of Gage's story, see http://www.deakin.edu.au/hbs/GAGEPAGE/Pgstory.htm.) "And that is what can happen when the neocortex is not functioning properly," Dr. Gamache said.

He also mentioned that sexual disinhibition can also occur with the deterioration of the neocortex. As I've already shared, Charles experienced significant sexual disinhibition later in his disease. When that was happening, Dr. Ravin explained that the actions weren't true to Charles's personality, but instead were the disease, and I tried to believe her. And the medication solutions she prescribed—adding the drug Seroquel and reducing the amount of Sinemet—seemed to work.

But throughout my grieving process, the memory of Charles's sexual disinhibition had haunted me. Had he really loved someone else instead of me during his last year or two of life? This thought was almost too painful to endure. Dr. Gamache's simple but scientific explanation cleared away my fear. The autopsy report confirmed that Charles's disease caused deterioration of the frontal lobe—and that would increase sexual disinhibition. The normal filters Charles would have used were broken. I'm indebted to Dr. Gamache for releasing me from mounting dismay.

SEEING CHARLES'S BRAIN CELLS

On what would have been our twenty-first anniversary, October 19, 2001, I had an appointment with the neuropathologist at McLean Hospital who had conducted Charles's autopsy a year and a half earlier. An elderly, articulate woman welcomed me into a small, cramped room that held a microscope, two swivel chairs, and shelves filled with small containers.

Ready for my visit, she had a neatly packed box of glass slides sitting on the counter. After our brief introductions, I explained that I wanted to understand Charles's autopsy report for the book I was writing. "His case was a difficult one to figure out, as it is hard to determine the difference between CBGD, PSP, or a variant of one with the other. While he had some clear signs of PSP, he also showed strong signs of CBGD. I even consulted with a colleague to make sure that my determination of CBGD was correct."

Then she pulled out the slides. She carefully placed one under the microscope, moving it to just the right spot before offering me the

chance to look. It took me a little while to adjust the focus and my eye
position so that I could see the cells smeared on the slide. "Do you see
the thin blue lines fanning across the slide from left to right with cells
scattered within?" she asked. I did. "That's good tissue with healthy
cells of the brain," she said. Then she moved the slide a bit, giving me
a different view, and asked, "Do you now see damaged cells arranged
in no particular pattern, no thin blue lines, just chaos? Those are the
diseased cells."

She continued with more samples, comparing the good cells with
the bad from various parts of Charles's brain. She showed me a
Milky Way of cells in a healthy section in contrast to a section with
very sparse cells. Other slides demonstrated healthy cells with clean,
clear shapes and a nucleus inside, as opposed to diseased cells shaped
like footballs and filled in with brown, or tangled with brown, or
yarnlike, or even cells that looked like brown sausages.

At the most minute level in Charles's brain, the cells that had
important functions—to coordinate his thinking, moving, and seeing—had been ravaged by his disease. His unusual symptoms developed because of these cellular-level changes.

Because of the autopsy, pieces of Charles's brain are now available
for scientists all over the world to learn more about CBGD. I left
McLean Hospital feeling awestruck at having been able to actually
see into Charles's brain. On that anniversary day, I had made one
more connection with Charles.

BUILDING AND MAINTAINING TRADITIONS

Charles maintained a number of traditions during our life
together. I didn't realize until after he died how important they had
been to me. Maybe they seem like little things, but now they bring
me tremendous fulfillment. And that has stimulated me to build a
few traditions of my own.

DOUGHNUT RUN
For years Charles took doughnuts and muffins to the Framingham

plant every Friday morning. He affectionately called it the doughnut run. It was his way of showing the front-line employees how much he appreciated their efforts. This tradition was so important to him that even when he was on vacation or on a business trip, he would recruit another Web manager to get the doughnuts for that Friday. He'd call the local Dunkin' Donuts early Friday morning to place his order. His phrasing was both consistent and endearing: "I'd like two dozen doughnuts and two dozen muffins, just mixed." Even when he could no longer drive and eventually was in a wheelchair, he continued to deliver the doughnuts each week.

October 14 approached—Charles's birthday, the first such commemoration after his death—and I pondered how to make the day special. I wanted to remind people of Charles. I got excited when I got the idea to repeat the doughnut run on the Friday of his birthday week.

The Friday morning of my first doughnut run in memory of Charles, I called Dunkin' Donuts and placed the order exactly as Charles had: "I'd like two dozen doughnuts and two dozen muffins, just mixed." But because I thought that the number of Web employees might have grown, I also ordered two dozen bagels as well. And I gave Charles's name for the order. When I got to Web to distribute the doughnuts, the employees expressed appreciation, shook my hand, asked how I was doing, thanked me, and shared that they missed Charles. I couldn't have asked for a more meaningful remembrance.

Anniversary Tradition

October 19, 2000—we would have celebrated our twentieth wedding anniversary the year Charles died. As with his birthday, I had planned in advance what I wanted to do to make the anniversary a memorable one and also, to create a new tradition for me. At the time, I had no idea what a roller-coaster day it would be.

The new tradition I had planned was to have dinner each year at a different restaurant that Charles and I had frequented. Then I would invoke the touching memory of Charles's gesture at our tenth anniversary: I would look through the folder that he'd saved that gave the chronology of our first year of dates, reminiscing about him and our marriage.

I started the anniversary day by keeping an annual appointment with my dermatologist. Just two weeks before, I had developed a small rash under my left arm and another small one on my back shoulder blade. Accompanying the rash was a numbness that radiated from my back around to my chest. The first thing the dermatologist said when I described my symptoms, before she even looked at the rash, was "Shingles." I had shingles! The condition is caused by a reactivation of herpesvirus, the cause of chicken pox that lies dormant in the bodies of those who have had the childhood disease. My body had finally succumbed to the abuse and stress of the last few years. The shingles explained why I had been so utterly fatigued.

When I arrived at work after the doctor's appointment, I held my biweekly staff meeting. What started out as a calm, orderly meeting quickly exploded into a personal conflict between two members of my staff, with one of them storming out of the meeting. Even though the two of them patched things up by the end of the day, the entire team's emotions, including mine, had been ratcheted up to high alert. The energy I needed for a quiet, pensive anniversary dinner that night was quickly waning.

Later in the day, I accompanied two staff members to a meeting with our new senior vice president. This was our first opportunity since his arrival at the company to meet with him and describe our team's illness prevention and wellness activities. We had no idea how he felt about our programs when we went in. But he lifted my spirits by showing his strong appreciation of our contribution to the company.

As the work day wound down, my exhaustion peaked. I vacillated about whether to follow through on my dinner plans. I just wanted to go home and go to bed. But then I thought of Charles, and that spurred me on. I had decided to go to a quaint Indian restaurant in Newton Center called India Paradise, located near the house where Charles and I had lived. We had loved the food and bread there. The last time we were there, Charles was in a wheelchair and Darry, his aide, had accompanied us.

Driving to Newton Center, I put on a Celine Dion CD and sobbed as our song, "Because You Loved Me," played. It finished just as I pulled up to our beautiful pink Victorian house that Charles had loved so much, but was now inhabited by new owners. I took out the small container of Charles's ashes that I had packed that morning and stood in front of the house, choking down the tears. I recited his touching mission, which I had memorized, and a poem that he used to say to me each night. Then, hoping that no one was aware, I tossed the ashes throughout the front garden.

I composed myself by the time I arrived at India Paradise. I enjoyed the delicious meal of chicken with lentils (and curry, of course) as well as baked naan. So many thoughts and memories came to me as I read through Charles's notes about every date he had listed, remembering where we went, what we did, and the important talks we'd had. For the first time in a number of years, I began to remember Charles as he was when he was well instead of his final years when he was incapacitated by disease.

This day of very high highs and low lows held some special kindnesses. My former boss, Sheila, brought me flowers in honor of my anniversary. I had had a chance to ride the train with her a few nights earlier, and she remembered the day. When I got home that night, I found that my friend Arlene, whom I had had dinner with the previous weekend, had left a voice message on my home phone to let me know that she had been thinking about me on my anniversary.

At the start of the meeting with my staff that morning, we had continued our tradition of reading a chapter out of Richard Carlson's book, *Don't Sweat the Small Stuff.* One of my staff members chose 90 when I asked someone to pick a number between 1 and 100, because that was how many chapters the book contained. "One More Passing Show" was the title of chapter 90. Ironically, that chapter described how the ups and downs of life all come and go. Life is just one thing after another—pain and pleasure. And each of these, the good and bad, will pass. Happiness comes when we allow ourselves, without struggling, to just go through the natural flow of everyday life. How apropos for the day I had!

CHRISTMAS TRADITION

I was standing in the checkout line at the local photocopy shop, having just made copies of some paperwork for my financial planner. Suddenly I noticed an advertisement for personalized calendars; just supply twelve pictures and store employees would assemble the calendar, the poster said. *Aha.* I had figured out how to make my Christmas holiday very special and to share that with my family.

At home, I rummaged through my pictures in search of a separate one of Charles with each of my family members. My favorite was the one that I used for July's page in the calendar, showing Charles and me with my mother at a July 4 celebration in Boston a few years earlier. Charles wore his Masada baseball cap. The small American flag we'd placed at the back of the cap stuck out brightly in the picture.

Some of the pictures dated back to earlier years in our marriage when we attended family reunions, holiday celebrations, or a funeral. The more current pictures included various family members on our trip to Russia and the Atlanta Olympics, as well as just hanging around our rented apartment or our new home. When I picked up the finished calendars, a warm, comfortable feeling flooded over me as I turned each page. The calendars turned out beautifully. Once I arrived home, I wrote in each person's name on his or her birth date on all eight calendars as a finishing touch.

Caregiving Affirmation:
Make it easier to get through difficult times by
creating traditions to memorialize your loved one.

I unveiled this gift of memory with my entire family, all twenty-three of them sitting around Carolyn's spacious family room after opening Christmas gifts. With everyone looking on, I flipped slowly through each page of one of the calendars, revealing each month's picture and the particular family members in it. "And thank you, everyone, for the unique support you each gave me and Charles during his illness," I said, fighting back tears.

I've continued this tradition each year since. Though the following year's calendars didn't focus solely on Charles, I have made sure that in each year's calendars, at least one month is devoted to Charles and another one to my father. The rest of the months capture magnificent memories of our family times together.

"I Love My Janet"

The most significant ritual that Charles started was a series of phrases he put together and recited to me every night as we went to bed.

It all started when Charles and I were first married. He frequently told me, "You're the best thing that ever happened to me." And whenever Gladys Knight's song "The Best Thing That Ever Happened to Me" came on the radio, he gave me a huge hug. These weren't just words for Charles. They expressed how he truly felt. He really made me believe that I was the best thing that ever happened to him.

Over time, he added on to that one phrase until it became an entire poem. And he got into the habit of repeating it to me each night as we snuggled together to go to sleep. "You're the best thing that ever happened to me" eventually grew into

> *I love my Janet. My pretty little gentle Janet.*
> *The love of my life is Janet my wife.*
> *I love you so, so, so, so, so much multiplied.*
> *I'm very proud of the person you are.*
> *The best thing that ever happened to me is you.*

The disease quickly stole Charles's ability to mentally put the words together, or to clearly speak them. I realized then that if we were to keep the ritual going, I would have to say it. So each night as he lay in bed, I would recite the words. I did that every night until the day he died.

My most prized possession is a sheet of paper on which Charles had typed the poem earlier in his disease. It was signed *Charles.* Looking at the squiggly lines of each letter of his name, it's obvious that he signed it with great difficulty.

After his death, I realized how much that little ceremony meant to me. It reminded me of how Charles skillfully made me feel good about myself. I couldn't let it die with him. I still recite it out loud when I go to bed. It is my way of remembering the meaning and self-esteem Charles brought to my life—and my ongoing connection with him.

E P I L O G U E

Scrounging through Charles's dusty old metal file cabinets, I discovered an autobiography he wrote on September 23, 1968, for his English 103 class while a freshman at Florida College in Tampa, a fundamentalist Christian institution. Mr. Garrett, the teacher, had scribbled an A in the top corner, and just below it, "Well done!"

My Life: The Quest for Greatness

Every small boy daydreams about the future, and I was no different. As a child, I anxiously awaited the time when I would grow to adulthood, dreaming of the great things that I would accomplish in my lifetime. Among my earliest recollections are those of strapping homemade guns and holsters around my waist as I rode across a fairyland prairie filled with outlaws and wild Indians. Cowboy boots and guns—to me these were glamorous; they symbolized greatness.

Later as my imagination was fed with a steady diet of adventure books and biographies of famous men, I began to picture myself in other facets of life. At one time I became a great soldier—a general leading his troops to victory over a desperate enemy. On another occasion I pictured myself as a great architect, erecting huge buildings for the world to exclaim at in awe and amazement. Yet again, at the height of my fantasies, I portrayed myself as the President of the greatest nation on earth, walking in the footsteps of George Washington and Abe Lincoln.

The story of my life is the tale of a quest for greatness—a search that grew and matured as a small child became a bigger boy and eventually a young man. I dreamed, as every child does, of being great—of seeking adventure and accomplishing great things.

I can recall few events of my early childhood. Vague impressions are all that remain of my earliest days. However, a few brief glimpses into the past stand out in my mind among the infinite maze of persons and places.

As a child, I became accustomed to moving vans, new houses, and strange people. My father is a preacher of the gospel, and thus my life has been one of beginning again every few years. Since the day nearly nineteen years ago when my parents tacked the name Charles Ralph Edmunson onto the small, red ball of noise that I later came to know as me, I have lived in eight communities in four different states. To a young boy, moving was a nightmare. There were the tears, the tearing of the heart, and the homesickness of a shy youth who was lost amid a sea of strange faces. However, the frequent changing of schools and friends was beneficial in the long run; it served as a challenge to me to prove myself to a new group of people.

Another aspect of my life—my cautious experiments into a foreign world of athletics—was prompted by a desire to make my Walter Mitty–like dreams of sports prowess into a reality. Quickly realizing, however, that I was too clumsy to dribble a basketball, and that I was too small to knock around on the football field, I turned to running for my varsity letters. Yet even at this I was not the athletic hero I had imagined myself as being. However, I ran my heart out; and despite my short legs, I finally developed to the point where I could call myself a member of the team. One of the happiest days of my youth came my junior year in high school when I proudly donned a white cross-country sweater with a big, red S on the front. That sweater eventually yellowed with age and was replaced by other, fancier sweaters and jackets, but that original one held a place in my heart that the others never reached.

Money played its role in my childhood as well. As a "preacher's kid," I learned early in life that a dollar was valuable—there were very few of them in our household. Consequently, I learned how to work in order to earn my spending money, and I discovered how to ease the family budget by buying some of my own clothes. Self-important in my industriousness, I went out on the streets at the age of ten selling newspapers. From this it was just a step to a paper route with its many responsibilities. During the summer I found that I could earn additional money by mowing yards and trimming hedges. Eventually at the age of fifteen, I found a job in a service station. Beginning as a helper who had never even checked the oil in a car, I progressed to the position of station manager with two other men looking to me for instructions. From this I turned to construction work, laboring with some bricklayers under the blistering sun.

From my parents I learned to save my money and to be frugal with my pennies. I was eleven years of age when I strutted to the bank, proudly bearing the first fifty dollars that I had earned and saved. This meager beginning formed the nucleus of a savings account that was to grow to finance my college education.

Early in life I developed an interest in the traditional American game of politics. A ten-year-old who comprehended very little of what was happening, I watched the Kennedy–Nixon debates in 1960, asking God in my childish prayers to help Nixon win the election. In 1964 I viewed with enthusiasm the rise of Barry Goldwater to popularity, and as November drew near, I crossed my fingers, hoping for the impossible. Two years later I crowed with delight as the Republicans recouped their losses. This set the background for my support of Nixon in the primaries and election of 1968.

One stigma that confronted me throughout childhood was the fact that my life was different from that of many of the people around me. During my early grades in school, I looked upon this as a reproach to me. I was unable to understand why my parents would not allow me to take part in dances or in Christmas celebrations as the other children did. When someone questioned my abstaining from these things, I was ashamed and embarrassed that I had to be unique.

When I became somewhat older, we moved to Searcy, Arkansas,

the most recent in a long chain of new homes. At this time my father left full-time preaching and went to work as a printer while he made plans to establish a conservative congregation in the heart of liberalism. This abrupt change shocked me into an awareness of the religion in which I had been reared. It became a family project to support the work of the new church. As I trudged from house to house delivering advertisements of services, and as I swept and prepared a room in a small union hall for services, I began to comprehend the full meaning of "Daddy's religion."

Several brief glimpses from the past come to mind, and I was able to sense them in a new perspective. I saw my father confronting an angry group of people with a piece of chalk and an open Bible. I recalled his driving nails late into the night as new classrooms were added to a small church building. I remembered a frightening debate where he sat calmly while another man shouted terrible things at him. I thought of the man in ragged clothes who returned to his family with a large sack of groceries after a talk with him.

Then I began to reexamine the values of the small child who had imagined himself to be a hero, performing feats which would have rivaled those of Superman. No longer was I embarrassed and tongue-tied when someone questioned my lack of conformity. I began to mature emotionally and spiritually as well as physically and mentally.

Resolving to be a gospel preacher, I took advantage of every opportunity to try out my newly found confidence. I became enthusiastic in Bible classes, and arguments at school on religious subjects became commonplace. My closest friends were besieged with tracts and lists of scriptures laboriously copied in a cramped, schoolboy hand.

Soon my first great opportunity came. Guthrie Dean, the evangelist from the church at Bald Knob, asked me if I would speak in his place on a Sunday evening. Consequently at the age of fourteen, I stood with trembling knees facing two hundred people and poured out my heart: "Millions of people are lost in sin . . . dying without a home. . . . The truth must be preached!"

Looking back, I can see that my first venture into the pulpit was no doubt a pitiful attempt; but rather than stifling my initiative, good and wise friends encouraged my feeble efforts. Before long, I received other invitations to speak, and eventually I began filling monthly appointments at two small rural churches.

In the meantime, about seventy-five conservative brothers began to meet in the VFW building at Newport, Arkansas, a city about fifty miles from my home. After they had been worshipping for six months, they called my father, asking him if I would preach for them the following Sunday. Since I did not have a driver's license at that time, my mother accompanied me to face these strange people. Although they had been expecting me to be somewhat older, the people complimented me on my efforts and asked me to speak again the next Sunday. Following this, I was invited to be their regular preacher. So as a junior in high school, I tacked the weekly preparation of two sermons onto my schedule of homework and track meets.

The nineteen months in which I preached at Newport were the richest of my life. There I baptized my first converts, and there also I discovered the awesome responsibilities of preaching the truth. I encountered opposition as I preached my convictions, and I learned how to defend my position as well as how to admit a mistake. This experience sharpened my appetite for proclaiming the Word rather than satisfying it.

Now I am a student at Florida College, endeavoring to prepare myself to be a more effective evangelist. Although I have grown considerably from the little boy who pictured himself as a great general, I still dream of being a great man. However, time and experience have changed the values of the small child to those of a young man standing on the threshold of adulthood.

I have reached the fulfillment of many of my earlier ambitions: I was chosen by my teachers as the most outstanding student; my classmates selected me to receive an award for citizenship; and I graduated as the valedictorian of my high school class. Yet as these and other honors fell my way, they seemed to be empty and meaningless, adding more disillusionment to my dissatisfaction with worldly standards of achievement.

I read in my Bible about another measure of greatness, which in the long run is vastly superior to the fantasies of a young boy. Jesus said: "He that is greatest among you shall be your servant . . . and whosoever shall humble himself shall be exalted." I have found a work that surpasses in greatness the achievements of the architect who erects huge skyscrapers or of the soldier who searches for adventure. James said: "He who converteth a sinner from the error of his way shall save a soul from death."

My quest for greatness has been redefined in a new dimension and laid out before me as a challenge. Only the future can tell how I will live up to it.

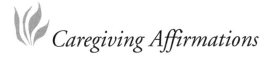 *Caregiving Affirmations*

CHAPTER 1

Approach your loved one sympathetically. A gentle approach
can bring breakthrough communication.

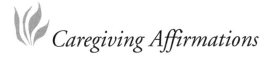

Engage actively with doctors to enhance your loved one's care.

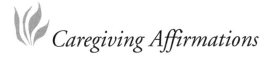

Reflect on your special relationship for inspiration
when life gets overwhelming.

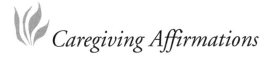

If you have the time and energy to do even a little research,
you and your loved one may feel a welcome sense of control
over the chaos of disease.

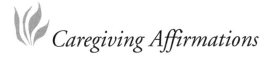

It's normal to feel shocked when you learn about
the severity of a neurodegenerative disease.

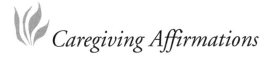

Explore the causes of the condition together to gain understanding.

Hold on to your passions, because they are the essence of who you are.

You'll be strengthened by continuing to work
toward your important goals.

Stay focused on what you enjoy.

Feel all of life's emotions.

CHAPTER 2

You can handle losses if you take them as they come.

When you respect each other's differences, you can overcome conflicts.

Use empathy to preserve your loved one's dignity.

Explore life's adventures together to store up
fond memories that will sustain you.

Actively work to minimize the feeling of being a victim.

Treatments won't always work. This isn't *your* failure.

Your loved one's struggles can bring out the best in you and in others.

Be creative and plan ahead when seeking ways
to ease difficult life transitions.

When you're faced with disappointments,
focus on at least one positive thing.

Use a symptom sheet to communicate more openly
with each other and your physicians.

Capitalize on opportunities as they arise and
as your loved one is ready for them.

*

A positive attitude will provide strength
to help you handle emotional pain.

*

CHAPTER 3

Despite your support, your loved one may still feel depressed.
Know that this is natural.

*

Use your creativity in finding solutions to new challenges.

*

Allow your loved one to maintain independence
in daily tasks as much as possible.

*

Take pleasure in every moment you spend together.

*

Expect caregiving demands to increase over time.

*

Find ways to include your loved one in events large and small.

Work together to make meaning out of the tragedy of disease.

Periodically reevaluate whether it's time to make major life changes.

No matter how overwhelmed you both are,
make a commitment to keep your spirits high.

Be aware that you'll win some and lose some
when trying new medical treatments.

You don't always have to be a fixer. Sometimes
your loved one needs only your empathy.

Be aware that your perspective may be very different
from your loved one's.

Because doctors are constantly making new discoveries,
consider taking a trip to the National Institutes of Health.

Accept that you won't be able to fix everything;
even creative solutions will sometimes fail.

❧

Look for the gifts that only this type of tragedy affords.

❧

Find fulfillment in persevering with your loved one.

❧

CHAPTER 4

Anticipate difficulty in finding dependable home health aides.

❧

Don't be shy about asking others for assistance.
Their willingness to help may astound you.

❧

Remember to enjoy the little things in life.

❧

A new world of freedom will open up once
your loved one agrees to use a wheelchair.

❧

Handling the most basic caregiving needs can be draining,
so seek the advice of experts to lighten your load.

Don't expect to always understand why your loved one
insists on certain things.

Prepare yourself for a diagnosis that may be devastating.

Embrace inspirational messages.

Live life to the fullest at every opportunity.

Watch for the warning signs of caregiver stress.

You'll be more at peace if you accept your loved one as is,
rather than futilely fighting the disease's symptoms.

Remember that difficult personality changes are
not your loved one—they are the disease.

CHAPTER 5

Provide opportunities for your loved one to hear accolades.

Give yourself credit for staying strong despite
being pushed to your limits.

Focus on the quality, not the length, of your loved one's life.

Consider hospice sooner versus later; the support will bring you relief.

Once you find the system that provides optimum help,
life can be much easier for you and your loved one.

Expect that some people will find it too difficult to visit
your loved one. That's okay—it doesn't mean that
they've stopped caring.

Let the love flow, even when all else is lost.

Plan to actively manage your aides—and learn from them, too.

Its perfectly normal to grieve even before your loved one dies.

Ease your burden by planning ahead for your loved one's death.

As long as your loved one hangs on, look for
reasons to hang on too.

Don't feel guilty in taking some time for yourself;
you need it to stay healthy.

A positive attitude can help get you through the toughest times.

CHAPTER 6

Being able to provide only palliative care and not curative care
can feel scary, but know that you are doing the best
you possibly can for your loved one.

It's okay to mourn what might have been.

❧

Expect the unexpected.

❧

You'll do friends and family members a kindness if you invite them to say their good-byes—but be prepared to mourn with them.

❧

Don't hide from your loved one's death. Open your heart to it, so that your loved one can let go more easily and so that you can begin to grieve in earnest.

❧

CHAPTER 7

Soak up the precious tributes to your loved one, who lives on through them.

❧

Know that if you welcome the waves of grief and the emotions that they evoke, you are helping yourself to heal.

❧

Consider an autopsy for your loved one to bring you peace of mind and the satisfaction of helping to further scientific knowledge.

❧

Make it easier to get through difficult times
by creating traditions to memorialize your loved one.

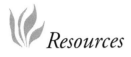 *Resources*

BOOKS

Albom, Mitch. *Tuesdays with Morrie.* New York: Doubleday, 1997.

Bloomfield, MD, Harold H., Melba Colgrove, PhD, and Peter McWilliams. *How to Survive the Loss of a Love.* New York: Bantam Books, 1983.

Carlson, Richard. *Don't Sweat the Small Stuff.* New York: Hyperion Books, 1997.

Frankl, Viktor. *Man's Search for Meaning.* New York: Pocket Books, 1997.

Hanh, Thich Nhat. *Touching Peace: Practicing the Art of Mindful Living.* Berkeley, CA: Parallax Press, 1992.

Kabat-Zinn, Jon. *Wherever You Go, There You Are: Mindfulness Meditation in Everyday Life.* New York: Hyperion Books, 1994.

Zonnebelt-Smeenge, Susan and Robert De Vries. *Getting to the Other Side of Grief: Overcoming the Loss of a Spouse.* Grand Rapids, MI: Baker Publishing Group, 1998.

ORGANIZATIONS

Brigham and Women's Hospital
A Harvard Medical school teaching affiliate
http://www.brighamandwomens.org

CBGD (Cortical Basal Ganglionic Degeneration) listserv
E-mail conversations with others interested in or suffering from CBGD
http://www.onelist.com/subscribe.cgi/cbgd_support

Harvard Brain Tissue Resource Center
Centralized resource for the collection and distribution of human brain specimens for brain research
http://www.brainbank.mclean.org

Massachusetts General Hospital
Harvard Medical School teaching affiliate
http://www.mgh.harvard.edu

McLean Hospital
Oldest neuropsychiatric research program in the United States
http://www.mclean.harvard.edu

MEDLINE
Database of medical journal articles
http://www.ncbi.nlm.nih.gov/entrez/query.fcgi

The Mind/Body Medical Institute, Chestnut Hill, MA
A program founded by Herbert Benson, MD, to help individuals with stress-related symptoms of chronic illness better manage their conditions.
http://www.mbmi.org

National Institute of Neurological Disorders and Stroke
Leading U.S. supporter of biomedical research on disorders of the brain and nervous system
http://www.ninds.nih.gov

National Institutes of Health
Health information, research, science education
http://www.nih.gov

National Library of Congress
Research, National Library Service for the Blind and Physically Handicapped, interpreting services (American Sign Language, contact signing, etc.)
http://www.loc.gov

National Organization for Rare Disorders
Information on research on rare diseases
http://www.rarediseases.org

Planetree Health and Healing Library
An organization in California connected with the Institute for Health &
Healing and the California Pacific Medical Center that conducts in-depth
MEDLINE searches for a fee
www.myhealthandhealing.org

The RIDE
Massachusetts' transportation service for the handicapped
http://www.mbta.com/traveling_t/disability_theride.asp
(For information about transportation services in other states, do an "all
states" search on the phrase handicapped transportation at
http://www.firstgov.gov)

Society for Progressive Supranuclear Palsy (PSP)
Education and support for those with PSP and their loved ones
http://www.psp.org/

University of Massachusetts Memorial Medical Center
Research and teaching hospital
http://www.umassmed.edu

U.S. National Library of Medicine
Health information, biomedical research, environmental health
http://www.nlm.nih.gov

Wayside Hospice, part of Parmenter Community Health
Special care for patients facing end of life issues by providing physical,
emotional, social and spiritual support for patients with a terminal diagnosis and their families.
http://www.parmenter.org

About the Author

Janet Edmunson took care of her husband, Charles, during the five years he fought a degenerative neurological disease. During that time, she also helped Charles write his book titled *Paradoxes of Leadership.* Janet has written a variety of articles, as well as chapters for books, including one titled "Precious Memories" in the book *Wise Women Speak: Changes Along the Path.*

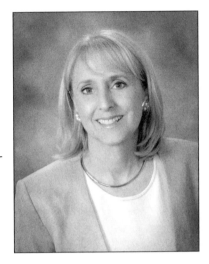

Janet has over thirty years' experience in the health promotion field and a master's degree in exercise science from Georgia State University. Leading the Prevention and Wellness staff of twenty at Blue Cross and Blue Shield of Massachusetts, Janet and her team support the company's promise to "always put our members' health first." The programs and initiatives she oversees encourage their 2.7 million members to adopt healthy lifestyles, support nearly 700 employers in offering worksite wellness programs for their employees, and provide tools to over 4,000 primary care physicians to promote preventative health.

Janet is also an inspirational speaker on leadership, health promotion, and caregiving.